1

ISBN: 9781077624436

SENIOR
FITNESS
Metric Edition

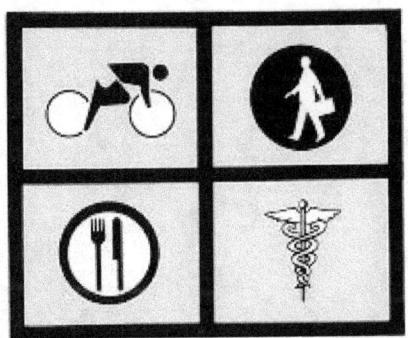

Vincent Antonetti, Ph.D.

NoPaperPress™

CONTENTS

LIST OF TABLES

LIST OF FIGURES

In most developed countries, people are living longer than ever before. But there's no getting around the fact that as we age, our bodies and minds change. Many older bodies often have several weakened systems. For many seniors their golden years are a life of restricted activity, of aches and pains – and visits to doctors. It doesn't have to be that way.

We can't stop the aging process. But what we do have some control over is whether, by our lifestyle and actions, we slow the process or speed it up. There are steps we can take to maintain our physical and mental capacity, measures that will allow us to live life to the fullest – and the longest. What is the secret? Most gerontologists agree that, in addition to doing something that is both mentally and emotionally rewarding, a **sensible**, regular physical exercise program and a nutritious diet are the keys. The fit senior typically has greater energy than his or her peers, does not get sick as often and is better able avoid chronic illnesses. In fact, a fit 70-year old can be as robust as a sedentary 35-year old. And it's never too late to start taking care of your body with exercise, proper nutrition and relaxation. This book presents the latest strategies to optimize your health and fitness in your golden years. You can have a better, actually a much better, quality of life. The time to start on your journey to fitness is now and the place to start is here.

What to Expect as You Age

Look in a mirror and you'll probably find a few more wrinkles and gray hairs – just a few of the changes you're likely to notice as you get older. The following is a list of other natural changes you can expect as you age.

Cardiovascular System Changes

Over time, your heart muscle becomes less efficient and has to work harder to pump the same amount of blood through your body. In addition, your blood vessels lose elasticity and fatty deposits may form on the inner walls of your arteries (atherosclerosis), narrowing the vessels. The natural loss of elasticity in combination with atherosclerosis makes your arteries stiffer, causing your heart to work even harder. All this can also lead to high blood pressure.

Bones, Muscles and Joint Changes

When you are about 30 years old, your bones reach their maximum mass. After that, your bones shrink in size and density. Gradual loss of density weakens your bones and makes them more susceptible to fracture. Aging causes the discs between your vertebrae to contract. As a consequence you might become shorter. In fact, people typically lose about 1 cm (0.4 inches) for every 10 years after age 40. And height loss is even greater after age 70. In total, you may lose 1 to 3 inches in height as you get older. Your muscles, tendons and joints also generally lose some strength and flexibility as you age.

Brain & Nervous System Changes

The number of cells (neurons) in your brain decreases with age, and your memory becomes less efficient. Your reflexes tend to become slower. You also tend to become less coordinated and may have difficulty with balance.

Urinary Tract Changes

As you age, your kidneys become less efficient at removing waste from your bloodstream. Chronic conditions such as diabetes or high blood pressure and some medications can damage your kidneys even further.

About one in 10 people age 65 and older experience a loss of bladder control (urinary incontinence). Women are more likely than men to have incontinence. Post-menopausal women might experience incontinence as the sphincter muscles around the opening of their bladder weaken, as bladder reflexes change, as the tissue lining their urethra becomes thinner and as pelvic muscles become weaker. In older men, incontinence is sometimes caused by an enlarged prostate, which can block the urethra. This makes it difficult to empty your bladder and can cause small amounts of urine to leak.

Eyes & Vision Changes

With age, your eyes may be less able to produce tears and your lenses gradually turn yellow and become less clear. As you know, in your 40s focusing on objects that are close up became more difficult and now you probably need reading glasses. Later, your pupils become less responsive making it more difficult to adapt to different levels of light. Other changes to your lenses can make you sensitive to glare, which presents a problem when driving at night. Familiar conditions that afflict seniors include cataracts, glaucoma and macular degeneration.

Ears & Hearing Changes

Hearing loss is one of the most common conditions affecting older adults and about half of all people older than age 85 experience significant hearing loss. Over the years, noises can damage the sensory hair cells of your inner ears. In addition, the walls of your auditory canals thin, and your eardrums thicken. You may have difficulty hearing high frequencies. Some seniors find it difficult to follow a conversation in a crowded room.

Dental Changes

Most adults retain their teeth throughout their lives. But how your teeth and gums respond to age depends on how well you've cared for them over the years. Even if you're meticulous about brushing and flossing, however, you may notice that your gums have receded and your teeth may darken slightly and become more brittle and break more easily. Some seniors experience dry mouth, which can lead to tooth decay and infection. Dry mouth can make speaking, swallowing and tasting difficult.

Skin Changes

With age, your skin thins and becomes less elastic and more fragile. You'll likely notice that you bruise more easily. Decreased production of natural oils may make your skin drier and more wrinkled. Age spots can occur, and small growths called skin tags are common. How fast your skin ages depends on many factors. The most significant factor is sun exposure over the years. The more sun your skin has been exposed to, the more damaged it may be. Smoking adds to skin damage in the form of wrinkles. Your risk of skin cancer also increases as you age.

Sleeping Pattern Changes

Your sleep needs change little as you get older. If you needed six hours of sleep when you were 25, chances are you'll always need six hours — give or take 30 minutes. However, as you age, you'll likely find that you sleep less soundly, meaning you'll need to spend more time in bed to get the same amount of sleep. By age 75, many people wake up several times each night.

Weight Changes

As you age, maintaining a healthy weight, or losing weight if you're overweight, may be more difficult. Your metabolism generally slows, meaning that your body burns fewer calories. Calories that were once used to meet your daily energy needs instead are stored as fat. In addition your level of activity may decrease, resulting in more unwanted pounds.

Sexuality Changes

With age, sexual needs, patterns and performance change. Women's vaginas tend to shrink and narrow, and the walls become less elastic. Vaginal dryness is a problem. All of this can make sex painful. Impotence becomes more common in men as they age. By age 65, as many as one in four men has difficulty getting or keeping an erection. In others, it may take longer to get an erection, and it may not be as firm as it used to be.

Senior Health Issues

According to the United States center for statistics, in 2007, the leading causes of death in U.S. seniors age 65 and older were cardiovascular disease (533,000 people), cancer (386,000), stroke (130,000) and diabetes (no data). That's the bad news. The good news is that research indicates that seniors who exercise regularly, who eat the right foods and who maintain a normal weight, i.e., who are physically fit, can reduce their risk of heart attack, stroke and diabetes, and also gain some protection against certain forms of cancer.

Heart Disease Risk Factors

Started in 1948, the "Framingham Study," under the direction of the National Heart Institute, examined thousands of people and demonstrated a clear statistical association between cardiovascular disease and a number of "risk factors." These risk factors have been found time and time again in the medical history of thousands of people who have had heart attacks.

Risk factors often attributed to our lifestyle and, therefore, under our control – at least to some extent – are in approximate order of importance:

1) Untreated high blood pressure.
2) Cigarette smoking.
3) High blood cholesterol.
4) Obesity.
5) Lack of physical activity.
6) A high-pressure existence.

No one of these factors has been called the single cause of cardiovascular disease. Indeed studies show that a combination of risk factors dramatically increases the danger.

Heart attack warning signs:

1) Prolonged, oppressive pain or unusual discomfort in the center of the chest. 2) Pain may spread to shoulder, arm, neck or jaw, and sweating, nausea, vomiting and shortness of breath may ensue.

Sometimes the symptoms subside, then return. If these warning signs are experienced, it is important to act quickly. If a doctor is not immediately available, get to a hospital emergency room at once.

Stroke & Warning Signs

Although some cells in the body can survive for as long as fifty minutes without blood, if the flow to the brain is cut off for ten or twenty seconds unconsciousness will occur, and deprived of blood circulation for four minutes or more results in brain damage. Blockage of the blood vessels leading to the brain or in the brain itself (sometimes a manifestation of atherosclerosis, other times caused by a clot) is called stroke. The warning signs are:

1) Sudden numbness or weakness of the face, arm or leg, especially on one side
2) Sudden headache, confusion, trouble speaking or understanding
3) Sudden trouble walking, dizziness, loss of balance or coordination
4) Sudden trouble seeing
5) Stroke and cardiovascular disease have a lot in common: High blood pressure is a major cause of both illnesses, and many of the preceding cardiovascular disease risk factors also apply to stroke.

Diabetes

With the ranks of the obese increasing dramatically, the incidence of diabetes is reaching epidemic proportions in the United States - posing a somber threat to our nation's well being. In 2010, diabetes was the fifth leading cause of non-accidental death in the United States. Type 2 diabetes is the most common form. Previously called adult-onset diabetes, type-2 diabetes can begin at any age. It usually starts with insulin resistance, a condition in which fat, muscle, and liver cells do not use insulin properly. **Being overweight and inactive (read unfit) increases your chance of developing type 2 diabetes.**

Counter Measures

It is not possible stop cardiovascular disease, heart attacks, stroke and diabetes completely, but enough is known to prevent many incidents. Be aware, however, that the battle against cancer is not as straight forward. Substantial evidence indicates a fit adult reduces their risk of cardiovascular disease, stroke, diabetes and only exhibits some benefit against certain malignances, such as colon cancer and breast cancer, and a promising benefit against others, but offers no protection with regard to many other cancers.

The physical conditions and living habits that increase the risk of premature heart disease, stroke and diabetes have been identified, but for every risk there is a counteracting step you can take. Said another way, to reduce your risk you need to look at your entire way of living and in some instances rearrange your priorities.

No one set of rules will guarantee health or fitness. Age, gender, and physical condition are all factors in determining the specific program that is best for you. We can delineate, however, the general guidelines for a total program:
1) Have periodic medical checkups.
2) Do not smoke.
3) Exercise regularly.

4) Practice good nutrition habits.

5) Maintain a proper weight level.

6) Learn to relax.

7) Drink alcohol in moderation.

In reality, it's a lot easier to prevent or delay many diseases and disabilities than it is to reverse damage from say a severe stroke, a debilitating heat attack, etc. The age-old adage "an ounce of prevention is worth a pound of cure" is certainly applicable to seniors looking to improve the quality of their life. In the pages that follow, a program will be outlined with a fitness prescription for seniors that is remarkably simple.

Benefits of Being Fit

While the results will differ from individual to individual, most often being fit most likely will result in a longer life expectancy, less illness, a healthful appearance, the ability to work (hey, most of us are retired) and play with vigor and an energy reserve for emergencies.

Seniors who start a physical fitness program and attain a heightened level of fitness, report a dramatic reduction in chronic fatigue, an improved ability to relax, more energy for day-to-day tasks, firmer muscles and increased strength. In short, they feel better – and look better too!

Staying physically active and exercising regularly can help prevent or delay many diseases and disabilities. In more specific terms, a well-designed total fitness program, encompassing exercise, nutrition and weight control, will:

1) Help you lose weight

2) Lower your blood pressure

3) Make your heart stronger

4) Keep your arteries supple

5) Speed up your basal metabolism

6) Convert fat to muscle

7) Make your muscles larger and stronger

8) Strengthen your bones

9) Improve your mood and often relieve symptoms of depression

Besides lowering your risk of heart disease, etc, being fit will also reduce your risk of injury due to falling (more on this later). In addition, according to the Harvard School of Public Health, your life expectancy increases about two hours for every hour of regular exercise. So we should add the following to our list of benefits of being fit:

10) You will look and feel younger than your chronological age

11) You will probably live longer

FITNESS ASSESSMENT

Before you begin your program, however, you should know where you stand, i.e., your current fitness level. Assessing your current level in areas such as aerobic (cardio) capacity, strength, flexibility, balance, percent body-fat, and even how appropriate your nutritional practices are, will help you establish what you should emphasize in your physical fitness program and help you set goals.

Medical Assessment

All seniors should have a medical assessment, or exam, before starting a physical fitness program. The medical checkup may be as simple as a visit to a physician who is familiar with your medical history, or it may be a thorough physical exam.

Note, in all cases the physician conducting the medical exam should be made aware of and should approve the specific physical fitness program you're planning. In addition, if you have or suspect you have cardiovascular disease or other health problems, if you are obese, if you have been totally inactive you should proceed with more care by having an exercising or stress-type EKG as part of your medical exam.

You can also get an indication of your overall condition by performing a few simple tests and taking some body measurements as outlined in the following pages.

Aerobic Assessment

A good measure of aerobic capacity, or cardio-respiratory fitness, is the volume of oxygen per minute per kilogram of body weight (called VO_{2max}) a person can process during hard exercise.

Higher values of VO_{2max} indicate better aerobic fitness. For example, a 25 year-old man in excellent physical condition can process about 50 milliliters of oxygen per minute per kilogram of body weight; compared to less than 20 mL/min/kg for a 70 year-old woman in poor condition.

One of the best self assessment tests for VO_{2max} is the Rockport Walking Test. This is a field test, not a laboratory test, and consists of walking one mile as rapidly as you can. At the end of the test you record your pulse and the time it took to complete the walk. You then convert the time to completion and your pulse into VO_{2max} using the formulae. Lastly, you enter Table 1 with your calculated VO_{2max} and determine your cardio-respiratory fitness level.

There is some risk if you take the Rockport Fitness Walking Test without prior conditioning. That is why the following precautions are strongly suggested.

1) Be sure to have a medical exam before taking the walking test.

2) Seniors should postpone the walking test until you have been exercising regularly for at least one month.

3) You must be able to comfortably walk at least two miles before you take the walking test.

When you take the test, if you feel exhausted, experience shortness of breath, become dizzy or light headed, or nauseous, stop the test. Do not attempt a retest until you have exercised regularly for at least another three months, when your fitness level should have improved.

One-Mile (1609 Meter) Walking Test

If available, walk on a school track or a measured and marked flat trail with a smooth surface. (Find an old one-quarter mile track and walk four laps on the inside lane for the one-mile test.) You also can use a treadmill rather than a track. Although not as accurate, if need be you can walk a street course you have driven and measured.

Before you start the test, warm up for several minutes with easy walking and stretching. Rest for about one minute. Then start the test. Walk as briskly as possible for one mile, but remember you'll probably walk at least 12 minutes, so don't start too fast. If you still feel strong, pick up the pace on the last lap.

When you finish the test, it's important to immediately measure your pulse. (Go to page 40 for recommended pulse measurement techniques.) At the conclusion of the test, you should feel slightly winded, but you should not be gasping for air. Your goal is to end the test feeling tired but not exhausted. Remember to cool down by continuing to walk slowly.

	Age	Cardio-Respiratory Fitness Level			
		Poor	Fair	Good	Excellent
Men	40-	30.2-	33.6-	39.0-	43.8-48.0
	50-	26.1-	31.0-	35.8-	41.0-45.3
	60-	20.5-	26.1-	32.3-	36.5-44.2
	70+	– No data –			
Women	40-	21.0-	24.5-	29.0-	32.9-36.9
	50-	20.2-	22.8-	27.0-	31.5-35.7
	60-	17.5-	20.2-	24.5-	30.3-31.4
	70+	– No data –			

Table 1: VO_{2max} versus Fitness Level

Calculating VO$_{2max}$: The following is undoubtedly the most difficult portion of this book, because VO$_{2max}$ is a function of so many variables: gender, weight, age, heart rate and time to complete the one-mile test walk. Although the formulae are relatively complex, we have tried to simplify the calculation as much as possible.

For women: VO$_{2max}$ = 133 – W – H – A – T

For men: VO$_{2max}$ = 139 – W – H – A – T, where

W = 0.17 × Weight (kg)

A = 0.39 × Age

H = 0.157 × Heart rate

T = 3.26 × Time to walk 1609 meters

Example: Determine VO$_{2max}$ and the fitness level of a 63 year-old man who weighs 70 kg. He finished the 1609 meter walking test in 14 minutes and 30 seconds (which is 14.5 minutes) with a heart rate of 130 beats per minute. The first step is to determine values for W, H, A and T.

W = 0.17 × Weight = 0.17 × 70 kg = 11.9

H = 0.157 × Heart rate = 0.157 × 130 = 20.4

A = 0.39 × Age = 0.39 × 63 years = 24.6

T = 3.26 × Time = 3.26 × 14.5 minutes = 50.5

Then calculate VO$_{2max}$ = 139 – W – H – A – T

VO$_{2max}$ = 139 – 11.9 – 20.4 – 24.6 – 50.5 = <u>31.6</u>

Finally, enter Table1 and find that a 63 year-old man with VO$_{2max}$ = 31.6, his fitness level is in the good category.

Strength Assessment

In the tests that follow you will use your own body weight to determine how strong you are. The standard tests are: the push-up test, the sit-up test, and the squat test. Because the sit-up test can aggravate existing lower back problems, we only recommend the push-up and squat tests. The objective in both tests is to see how many push-up and squat repetitions you can perform without stopping.

Push-up Test: For the test, men should execute the standard military push-up; i.e., your back and trunk should be rigid and straight and your weight should be supported by your arms and toes. Women should employ the familiar half push-up, supporting their weight with their arms and knees. Use Table 2 to assess your performance.

Gender	Age	Push-up Performance		
		Below Average	Average	Above Average
Men	40-	5 - 14	15 - 24	25 - 29
	50-	0 - 9	10 - 19	20 - 24
	60-	0 - 4	5 - 9	10 - 15
	70+	0 - 1	2 - 4	5 - 8
Women	40-	0 - 7	8 - 19	20 - 29
	50-	0 - 5	6 - 14	15 - 23
	60-	0 - 2	3 - 5	6 - 8
	70+	– No data –		

Table 2: Push-up Test

Squat Test: Stand about 30 cm in front of a chair. Place your feet about shoulder width apart and extend your arms parallel to the floor to your front. Bend your knees and slowly lower your body until your butt just touches the seat of the chair. (But don't sit on the chair.) Then slowly return to the standing position. Repeat as often as you can without stopping. Use Table 3 to assess your performance.

Gender	Age	Squat-Test Performance		
		Below Average	Average	Above Average
Men	40-	18 - 20	21 - 23	24 - 26
	50-	15 - 17	18 - 20	21 - 23
	60-	12 - 14	15 - 17	18 – 20
	70+	– No data –		
Women	40-	12 - 14	15 - 17	18 - 20
	50-	9 - 11	12 - 14	15 - 17
	60-	6 - 8	9 - 11	12 - 14
	70+	– No data –		

Table 3: Squat Test

Flexibility Assessment

The sit and reach test is a standard way to determine hip and trunk flexibility and is often used as a measure of overall flexibility.

Sit & Reach Test: Remember to warm up with a few gentle stretches before you start the test. First tape a meter stick to the floor at the 23-cm mark. Remove your shoes and sit on the floor, with your legs forward and fully extended, so that the meter stick is between and almost parallel to your extended legs. (The meter stick's zero mark should be closest to you). Locate your heels at the 23-cm mark and move your feet about 25 cm apart. Place one hand over the other and slowly stretch forward (without jerking or bouncing), and extend the tips of your fingers as far as possible along the meter stick. Repeat three times. Your score is the furthest or highest number you are able to reach. Use Table 4 to assess your flexibility.

Gender	Age	Sit & Reach-Test Performance		
		Below Average	Average	Above Average
Men	40-	9.0 -	12.5 -	16.1 -
	50-	8.5 -	12.0 -	15.6 -
	60-	6.0 - 9.9	10.0 -	14.1 -
	70+	– No data –		
Women	40-	10.0 -	14.5 -	19.1 -
	50-	10.0 -	14.5 -	17.6 -
	60-	10.0 -	14.0 -	17.1 -
	70+	– No data –		

Table 4: Flexibility - Sit & Reach

Balance Assessment

As people grow older, many have difficulty with their balance. Balance disorders are one of the main reasons why older people fall. An assessment of your balance and your the risk of falling can be obtained by completing the following simple self-administered questionnaire.

The ABC Balance Confidence Scale: For each of the following situations indicate your level of confidence in doing the activity without losing your balance or becoming unsteady. Choose a percentage on the ABC rating scale from 0% confident to 100% confident. How confident are you that you will <u>not</u> lose your balance or become unsteady when …

1) Walk around the house?
2) Walk up or down stairs?
3) Bend over & pick up a slipper from the floor?
4) Reach for an item on a shelf at eye level?
5) Stand on tiptoes & reach for an item above your head?
6) Stand on a chair and reach for something?
7) Sweep the floor?
8) Walk outside the house to a parked car?
9) Get into or out of a car?
10) Walk across a parking lot to a mall?
11) Walk up or down a ramp?
12) Walk in a crowded mall with people walking past you?
13) Get bumped by people as you walk in a mall?
14) Step on or off an escalator while holding onto a railing?
15) Step on or off an escalator while not holding a railing?
16) Walk outside on icy sidewalks?

(If you do not currently do an activity in the questionnaire, try and imagine how confident you would be if you had to do the activity) . If you normally use a walking aid to do the activity or hold onto someone, rate your confidence as if you <u>were not using</u> these supports.

For each question your answer should consist of a whole number (0 to 100%). Add all your answers (possible range = 0 to 1600) and divide by 16 to get your ABC score. Use Table 5 to assess your balance and your risk of falling.

ABC Score	Interpretation
80 to 100%	High functioning level
50 to 80%	Moderate functioning
0 to 50%	Low functioning level
66% or less	**High risk of future fall**

Table 5: The ABC Balance Assessment

Body-Weight Assessment

Recently, many health-care practitioners rely on Body Mass Index, or BMI, to determine if a person is overweight. The BMI takes into account both a person's weight and height and is calculated by dividing a person's weight in kilograms by the square of their height (in meters). Table 6 provides a convenient determination of BMI. This table would not be applicable to competitive athletes, body builders and the chronically ill.

Weight (kg.)	- Height (cm.) -									
	155	160	165	170	175	180	185	190	195	200
45	18.7	17.6								
50	20.8	19.5	18.4							
55	22.9	21.5	20.2	19.0	18.0					
60	25.0	23.4	22.0	20.8	19.6	18.5	17.5			
65	27.1	25.4	23.9	22.5	21.2	20.2	19.0	18.0		
70	29.1	27.3	25.7	24.2	22.9	21.6	20.5	19.4	18.4	17.5
75	31.2	29.3	27.5	26.0	24.5	23.1	21.9	20.8	19.7	18.8
80	33.3	31.2	29.4	27.7	26.1	24.7	23.4	22.2	21.0	20.0
90	37.5	35.2	33.1	31.1	29.4	27.8	26.3	24.9	23.7	22.5
100	41.6	39.1	36.7	34.6	32.7	30.9	29.2	27.7	26.3	25.0
120	49.9	46.9	44.1	41.5	39.2	37.0	35.1	33.2	31.6	30.0
140			51.4	48.4	45.7	43.2	40.9	38.8	36.8	35.0
160				55.4	52.2	49.4	46.7	44.3	42.1	40.0
180						55.6	52.6	49.9	47.3	45.0

Table 6 Body Mass Index (BMI)

BMI	Weight Profile
18.5 or less	Underweight
18.6 to 24.9	Normal
25.0 to 29.9	Overweight
30.0 to 39.9	Obese
40 or more	Extremely Obese

Table 7 Weight Profile vs. BMI

The rationale behind the BMI is based on epidemiological data that show an increase in mortality when the BMI is above 25, although the increase in mortality tends to be moderate until a BMI of 30 is reached. Table 7 shows how a person's body-weight is categorized as a function of BMI.

BMI-Based Weight vs. Height

Another more convenient way to use BMI is the **New** BMI-Based Weight vs. Height Chart shown in Table 8, where the underweight category corresponds to BMI = 18.5 or less, normal weight is for BMI = 18.6 to 24.9, overweight is for BMI = 25.0 to 29.9, obese is for BMI = 30.0 to 39.9 and extremely obese is for BMI = 40 or more.

Table 8 BMI-Based Weight (kg) vs. Height

Height (cm)	Normal Range	Overweight Range	Obese Range
150	41.9 – 56.0	56.1 – 67.3	67.4 – 89.8
152	43.0 – 57.5	57.6 – 69.1	69.2 – 92.2
154	44.1 – 59.1	59.2 – 70.9	71.0 – 94.6
156	45.3 – 60.6	60.7 – 72.8	72.9 – 97.1
158	46.4 – 62.2	62.3 – 74.6	74.7 – 99.6
160	47.6 – 63.7	63.8 – 76.5	76.6 – 102.1
162	48.8 – 65.3	65.4 – 78.5	78.6 – 104.7
164	50.0 – 67.0	67.1 – 80.4	80.5 – 107.3
166	51.3 – 68.6	68.7 – 82.4	82.5 – 109.9
168	52.5 – 70.3	70.4 – 84.4	84.5 – 112.6
170	53.8 – 72.0	72.1 – 86.4	86.5 – 115.3
172	55.0 – 73.7	73.8 – 88.5	88.6 – 118.0
174	56.3 – 75.4	75.5 – 90.5	90.6 – 120.8
176	57.6 – 77.1	77.2 – 92.6	92.7 – 123.6
178	58.9 – 78.9	79.0 – 94.7	94.8 – 126.4
180	60.3 – 80.7	80.8 – 96.9	97.0 – 129.3
182	61.6 – 82.5	82.6 – 99.0	99.1 – 132.2
184	63.0 – 84.3	84.4 – 101.2	101.3 – 135.1
186	64.3 – 86.1	86.2 – 103.4	103.5 – 138.0
188	65.7 – 88.0	88.1 – 105.7	105.8 – 141.0
190	67.1 – 89.9	90.0 – 107.9	108.0 – 144.0
192	68.6 – 91.8	91.9 – 110.2	110.3 – 147.1
194	70.0 – 93.7	93.8 – 112.5	112.6 – 150.2
196	71.5 – 95.7	95.8 – 114.9	115.0 – 153.3
198	72.9 – 97.6	97.7 – 117.2	117.3 – 156.4
200	74.4 – 99.6	99.7 – 119.6	119.7 – 159.6

Example: Determine BMI of a man who is 190 cm tall and weighs 80 kg. First use Table 6. Scan the far left of the table and locate his weight of 80 kg. From this number run your finger horizontally (to the right) until it intersects the vertical column headed by his 190 cm height. The number at the intersection is his BMI = 22.2. According to Table 7 his weight is in the normal range.

Example: Determine the "normal" (healthy) weight range for a man who is 190 cm tall. From Table 8, find that at 190 cm he must weigh between 67.1 and 89.9 kg for his weight to be in the "normal" range, that is for his BMI to be between 18.6 and 24.9. (I think you will agree that Table 8 provides information that is more useful than does Table 6.)

Waist-to-Hip Ratio: Another important weight-profile parameter is your waist-to-hip ratio. Health risks for heart attack and stroke increase considerably for:
   - Men with a waist to hip ratio greater than 1.0.
   - Women with a waist to hip ratio greater than 0.8.
To calculate your ratio, measure your waist size (at its narrowest circumference) and divide it by your hip size (at the widest section). For example, a man with a 110-cm waist and 90-cm hips would have a waist to hip ratio of 110/90 = 1.2, and would have an increased risk for health problems.

Nutrition Practices Assessment
Nutrition is not normally part of a fitness assessment, but it's included here because it's a crucial and often overlooked element of a comprehensive physical fitness program. To broadly assess how appropriate your current nutritional practices are please complete the following questionnaire.
a) Vegetable servings eaten per day?
None (1 point), 1 serving (2 points), 2 to 4 (3 points), 5 or more (4 points)
b) Fruit servings eaten per day?
None (1 point), 1 serving (2 points), 2 to 4 (3 points), 5 or more (4 points)
c) Cereal & whole-grain bread servings per day?
None (1 pt), 1 serving (2 pts), 2 to 4 (3 pts), 5 or more (4 pts)
d) How many times per week do you eat a fish or poultry?
Never (1 pt), 1 time (2 pts), 2 to 3 (3 pts), 4 or more (4 pts)
e) How do you prepare and eat poultry?
Fry dark meat with skin & gravy (1 pt)
Bake or broil dark meat with skin & gravy (2 pts)

Bake or broil dark meat without skin (3 pts)
Bake or broil white meat without skin (4 pts)
f) How many times per week do you eat beans, lentils, peas?
Never (1 pt), 1 time (2 pts), 2 to 3 (3 pts), 4 or more (4 pts)
g) How often per week do you eat burgers, frankfurter, bacon, etc?
7 or more (1 pt), 4 to 6 (2 pts), 2 to 3 (3 pts), Rarely (4 pts)
h) When you consume milk, yogurt, ice cream, etc, you most often select:
Only whole-fat dairy product (1 pt)
Whole milk, but low-fat yogurt & ice cream (2 pts)
Low-fat (1 or 2% fat) (3 pts)
Skim or non-fat products (4 pts)
i) If ordering potatoes in a restaurant would you choose:
French fried or hash brown (1 pt)
Baked or boiled with butter and/or sour cream (2 pts)
Boiled without butter or sour cream (3 pts)
Baked without butter or sour cream (4 pts)
j) How many times per week do you eat fast-food?
5 or more (1 pt)
3 or 4 times (2 pts)
1 or 2 (3 pts)
Rarely (4 pts)
k) Do you add salt to your food?
At every meal (1 pt)l
Once per day (2 pts)
2 or 3 times per week (3 pts)
Rarely (4 pts)
l) How often do you eat sweets (cookies, candy bar, etc)?
More than one sweet per day (1 pt)
About one per day (2 pts)
2 to 4 sweets per week (3 pts)
Rarely (4 pts)
m) Do you take any vitamin or mineral supplements?
None (1 pt)
Take herbal supplements (2 pts)
Take individual vitamins (like C, E, etc) (3 pts)
Take multi-vitamin & mineral supplement (4 pts)
n) If you want to lose weight, how do you proceed?
Go on a crash die (1 pt)
Stop eating carbs (2 pts)

Cut back on carbs & increase exercise (3 pts)
Reduce caloric intake & increase exercise (4 pts)

This completes our brief nutrition practices assessment. Add up your score and see how you compare to the following standards.

Excellent = 49 to 56 points
Good = 41 to 48
Fair = 32 to 40
Poor = 23 to 31
Very Poor = 14 to 22

Time to Set Goals

Now it's time to review your fitness-self-assessment test results and set some broad personal fitness goals, such as losing weight and improving your aerobic capacity. You're not quite ready to construct a total program. That will have to wait until you read the exercise, nutrition and weight control chapters. These topics are somewhat complex and are treated in depth in the pages that follow.

IMPROVE YOUR BALANCE

An intact sense of balance helps you walk without staggering, get up from a chair without falling and climb stairs without tripping. But as we age changes, such as diminished balance and weakened depth perception, often occur that can make falls more likely. In fact, accidents are the sixth leading cause of death in persons over age 75, with falls being the leading reason. Each year, 1.8 million Americans over age 65 are injured in falls. Many factors contribute toward making an older adult susceptible to falls. These include: impaired hearing and vision, general loss of muscular strength and tone, arthritis, vertigo (the feeling that you or the things around you are spinning), cerebral-vascular insufficiency, neurologic disability (stroke), changes in spinal alignment, sudden decrease in blood pressure as you stand and various illnesses such as Parkinson's disease.

Balance Disorders

There are many types of balance disorders. One of the most common is benign paroxysmal positional vertigo (BPPV). With BPPV, you experience a relatively brief, but intense feeling of vertigo that can occur when you change the position of your head. You may also experience BPPV when you roll over to your left or right in bed, or as you get out of bed in the morning, or when you look up at an object on a high shelf. In BPPV, small calcium deposits in the inner ear become displaced, causing a person to feel dizzy. The cause of BPPV is not known, although it may be caused by an inner ear infection, head injury, or just aging.

Labyrinthitis is an infection or inflammation of the inner ear that causes dizziness and loss of balance. The labyrinth is the organ in your inner ear that helps you maintain your balance.

Ménière's disease is a another balance disorder. The symptoms include vertigo, hearing loss that comes and goes, tinnitus (a ringing or roaring in the ears) and a feeling of fullness in the ear.

Balance disorder treatment options depend on the cause. For example, if caused by medication, your doctor may change the type of medication or lower the dosage. And BPPV can be treated by manipulating the head (moving the calcium deposits to a position where they don't cause problems).

Reduce Your Risk of Falling

In 2010, the last year for which statistics are available, 433,000 people over 65 were admitted to hospital after falling, and a shocking 15,800 died as a direct result of the fall. Less visible are the many who survive a fall but suffer indirect consequences – including pneumonia, infection, muscle loss, etc. Once considered an inevitable part of aging, falls are now recognized as complex, often preventable events with multiple causes and consequences. The following multi-pronged approach can greatly reduce your chances of falling.

Trip-proof Your Home: Tour your home for anything that could cause you to trip. Area rugs and electric cords are notorious hazards. You're more likely to lose your balance in a dark space because you don't have a spatial point of reference. So add brighter lighting, and install night-lights in hallways and bathrooms so you don't stumble if you get up in the middle of the night. Place non-slip mats on shower and bathtub floors. Consider adding grab bars next to and inside your shower or tub

Get a Medication Check-Up: Have a health care provider review of all your medications including nonprescription drugs like supplements and cold medicines. Drug interactions or side effects such as drowsiness or dizziness can make falls more likely.

Have Your Vision Checked: Schedule a vision check because poor vision or eyesight clouded by cataracts or glaucoma can also increase your chances of falling.

Strengthen Your Legs: Exercise improves leg strength which in turn can reduce your risk of falling. The ideal time for someone to begin an exercise program is before you have a fall. But it's never too late.

Walking, stretching, weight training, dancing, yoga, and tai chi can improve mobility and balance – even after a fall. In addition to making daily life a lot easier, strong legs can also help catch you if you do trip. The easiest way to strengthen your legs is to use them more. Walk around the block. Take the stairs. Practice standing up and sitting down from a chair. Work in your yard. Anything that uses your legs will make them a bit stronger.

Train Your Balance: Few seniors know that you can train your balance. Balance exercises involves putting your body into a slightly unstable position. This can include standing with one foot in front of the other like you're on a balance beam, or standing on one foot. Just place your feet in the correct position and try to hold for ten to twenty seconds. You should always do balance exercises next to something that you can hold on to if you need to, like a sturdy chair, table, doorknob or the back of a couch. Balance exercises can be done daily.

Balance Training Exercises

The following are specific exercises designed to improve your balance. Once again remember to initially hold onto a secure object when performing balance exercises.

a) Plantar Flexion Exercise (See Figure 1 on next page)
1) Stand straight, holding onto a table or chair for balance.
2) Slowly stand on tip toe, as high as possible.
3) Hold this position.
4) Slowly lower heels all the way back down.
5) Repeat 8 to 15 times.
6) Rest a minute, then do another 8 to 15 repetitions.
7) As you progress, hold onto the chair with one hand, then one fingertip, then no hands and finally, if you are steady, with your eyes closed.

b) Knee Flexion Exercise
1) Stand straight; hold onto table or chair for balance.
2) Slowly bend one knee up as far as possible, so your foot is behind you.
3) Hold this position.
4) Slowly lower your foot all the way back down.
5) Repeat with other leg.
6) As you progress, hold onto the chair with one hand, etc.

c) Hip Flexion Exercise
1) Stand straight; holding onto a table or chair for balance.
2) Slowly bend one knee toward chest, without bending waist or hips.
3) Hold this position.
4) Slowly lower your leg all the way down.
5) Repeat with other leg.
6) As you progress, hold onto the chair with one hand, etc.

d) Hip Extension Exercise
1) Stand 12 to 18 inches from table.
2) Hold onto a chair and bend slightly at hips.
3) Slowly lift one leg straight backwards.
4) Hold this position
5) Slowly lower leg.
6) Repeat with other leg.
7) As you progress, hold onto the chair with one hand, etc.

e) Side Leg Raise Exercise

1) Stand straight - directly behind a table or chair, feet slightly apart.
2) Hold onto chair for balance.
3) Slowly lift one leg to side, 6-12 inches.

e) Side Leg Raise Exercise

1) Stand straight - directly behind a table or chair, feet slightly apart.
2) Hold onto chair for balance.
3) Slowly lift one leg to side, 6-12 inches.
4) Hold position.
5) Slowly lower leg.
6) Repeat with other leg.

Note: Your back and knees are straight throughout the exercise.
As you progress, hold onto the chair with one hand, etc.

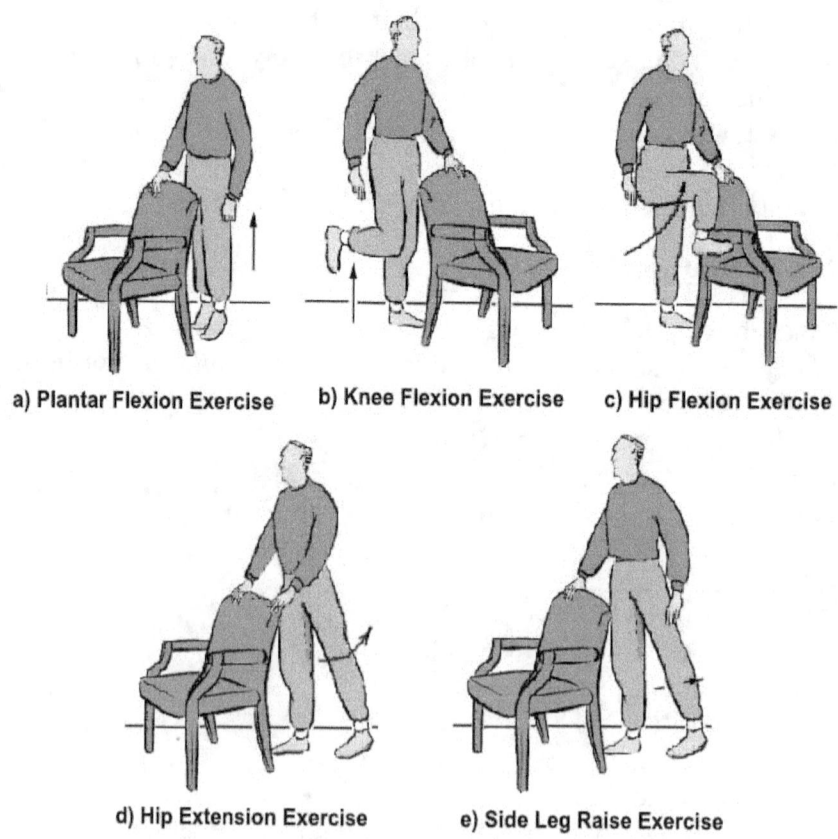

a) Plantar Flexion Exercise   b) Knee Flexion Exercise   c) Hip Flexion Exercise

d) Hip Extension Exercise   e) Side Leg Raise Exercise

Figure 1: Balance Training Exercises

Anytime/Anywhere Exercises

These exercises can also improve your balance. Do them almost anytime, anywhere, and as often as you like, as long as you have something sturdy nearby to hold onto if you become unsteady.

1) Walk heel-to-toe. Position your heel just in front of the toes of the opposite foot each time you take a step. (Your heel and toes should touch or almost touch.)

2) Stand on one foot (while waiting in line at the grocery store or at the bus stop, for example). Alternate feet.

3) Stand up and sit down. Try to gradually decrease use of your arms as your legs as you get stronger.

EXERCISE FOR SENIORS

For most people, the common tasks of living and working no longer provide enough exercise to develop and maintain cardiovascular and respiratory fitness and good muscle tone. But the bodies we inherited are just not built to be immobile and passive. There are two ways to become more physically active: 1) Increase the physical activity in your daily life; and 2) Start on a regular exercise program. Better still would be a combination of both.

Be More Active Every Day

Before we address exercise programs, here are some ways you can increase physical activity in your daily routine: First, change your attitude toward the occasional "bothersome" physical tasks that you encounter in daily living. Consider anytime you have to lift, bend, reach, walk, as an opportunity to burn additional calories and as an extension of your formal workout. Look for opportunities to walk, such as walking up stairs (two at a time if you can) rather than using an elevator, walking to a local store rather than driving, walking the course if you play golf, and mowing your lawn. At work stand up and stretch two or three times a day, read standing up, etc. Engage in leisure activities such as dancing, bowling and gardening more often. Each of these daily activities taken alone may not seem like much, but done every day for many years they can add up to a substantial number of extra calories burned.

Calories Burned

Table 9 (on the following page) shows the number of calories burned per hour for various activities. Notice that the calories expended for a given activity depends on your weight. Good news: **For any activity, the more you weigh the more calories you burn!**

Example: Determine the number of kcalories burned by a 86 kg man (or woman) who walks 11 kilometers in two hours.

First calculate the person's walking speed = 11 km / 2 hours = 5.5 kph. Because 86 kg is not listed in Table 9, we use the neighboring value of 90 kg. Then from Table 9, we find walking at 5.5 kph, a 90 kg person burns 392 kcalories per hour. Thus, in two hours a 90-kg person would burn 2 x 392 = 784 kcal.

But from this we must subtract the number of kcal a 90 kg person would have used anyway if, instead of walking, he or she just sat for the two hours. From Table 9 this amounts to 115 kcal per hour, or 230

kcalories in two hours. Then the net energy a 90 kg person would expend walking (over and above just sitting) totals 784 – 230 = 554 kcal.
But the individual in this example weighs 86 kg and would expend fewer calories than a 90 kg person: 554 x 86/90 = **529 kcal**

Activity	Weight (kg)								
	50	60	70	80	90	100	110	120	130
Aerobics (dance)	450	540	630	720	810	900	990	1080	1170
Basketball	350	420	490	560	630	700	770	840	910
Bicycling (20 kph)	400	479	559	639	719	799	879	959	1039
Cycling (in place)	350	420	490	560	630	700	770	840	910
Calisthenics	313	375	438	500	563	625	688	750	813
Cricket	250	300	350	400	450	500	550	600	650
Dancing	229	275	321	366	412	458	504	550	595
Football	376	451	526	602	677	752	827	902	978
Golf (pulling cart)	248	297	347	396	446	495	545	594	644
Golf (riding cart)	174	209	244	278	313	348	383	418	452
Handball	335	402	469	536	603	670	737	804	871
Hiking	294	352	411	470	528	587	646	704	763
Horseback riding	197	236	276	315	355	394	433	473	512
Jogging (12 kph)	624	748	873	998	1122	1247	1372	1496	1621
Mowing lawn	275	329	384	439	494	549	604	659	714
Raking leaves	301	361	421	482	542	602	662	722	783
Rowing (moderate)	349	418	488	558	627	697	767	836	906
Sitting	64	77	90	102	115	128	141	154	166
Skating	349	418	488	558	627	697	767	836	906
Skiing (+ country)	399	479	559	638	718	798	878	958	1037
Skiing (downhill)	303	363	424	484	545	605	666	726	787
Squash	335	402	469	536	603	670	737	804	871
Swimming laps	404	484	565	646	726	807	888	968	1049
Tennis (singles)	294	352	411	470	528	587	646	704	763
Tennis (doubles)	223	267	312	356	401	445	490	534	579
Walking 4.8 kph	178	214	249	285	320	356	392	427	463
Walking 5.5 kph	218	262	305	349	392	436	480	523	567
Walking 6.5 kph	277	332	388	443	499	554	609	665	720

Table 9: Calories Burned for Various Activities

31

Types of Exercise

Simply stated there are **three basic types of exercise: aerobic, stretching, and strengthening**.

Aerobic exercises (also called "cardio") condition your cardiovascular system. Aerobic exercises, such as jogging, swimming, cycling, brisk walking, skipping rope, jogging in place, and many others, are typically deep breathing and continuous, with rhythmic and repetitive contractions of your large muscle groups. The main goal of an aerobic exercise program is to increase the rate which your body can process oxygen, i.e., increase VO_{2max}. A well-conditioned person with efficient lungs and a strong heart can pump large volumes of blood, can breathe large volumes of air, and via the blood circulatory system effectively transport the oxygen in the air they breathe to all parts of their body.

Regular aerobic exercise "trains" the heart to pump more blood with less effort. Aerobic exercise improves the circulatory system by developing more elastic arteries and by creating peripheral or extra blood paths to the heart; and aerobic exercise strengthens the muscles of respiration increasing the volume of oxygen that can be processed within a given time. Done regularly, aerobic exercises improve stamina and endurance, and most importantly promote what should be your central exercise goal - cardiovascular fitness. For if your cardiovascular system is not in shape, you're not in shape - no matter how many push-ups or crunches you can do!

Stretching-type exercises such as yoga, tai chi, Pilates and to a lesser extent calisthenics can improve your flexibility – and some of the exercises can make you somewhat stronger.

As you age you inevitably start to loose flexibility. Your gait becomes stiffer; you can't stand quite as upright as you used to; it becomes tougher to bend over; and you have difficulty turning your neck. Regardless of your age, however, stretching can make you more flexible, less injury prone, and can
reduce the pain and discomfort associated with tight muscles and shortened tendons. Realize, however, that stretching exercises do not condition your heart and lungs. Stretching exercises are fine as long as they are performed in addition to rather than in place of an aerobic exercise.

Most experts do recommend stretching before and after aerobic and strength routines. However, never stretch cold muscles and always do some form of warm up prior to stretching. Stretch slowly and hold gently. You should stretch to the point of feeling a mild pull, but you should never feel pain. And when you stretch – do not bounce.

Muscle and strength **building exercises,** e.g., weight lifting, use of the machines found in fitness centers and isometrics.

Once more, as you age you loose muscle mass, your bone density decreases and you lose strength. Exercises like weight lifting strengthen your muscles, bones and joints. Strengthening exercises also reduce your risk of developing osteoporosis, a severe bone-loss disease, which can lead to easily fractured bones and all the complications that often follow. Strong muscles not only allow you to lug groceries up to a second floor apartment, but as with increased flexibility, strong muscles also make you less injury prone. **Strengthening exercises are beneficial and should be a part of your fitness routine, but again they should be performed in addition to an aerobic exercise** because alone they cannot condition your heart and lungs.

Select the Right Exercise

Selecting the right fitness exercise is the key to a successful conditioning program. You should try to pick an activity (or activities) you will enjoy. You may decide to concentrate on one activity such as squash, or you may choose to walk briskly some days and lift weights on other days.

Incidentally, three to five days of a vigorous aerobic exercise plus two days of either strength or flexibility exercises per week is a good combination. Whatever you settle on make sure it is an activity (or activities) that can be done regularly and that you enjoy. Factors to consider in choosing your activity are:

Your Medical Condition: If you have a medical condition such as a heart problem, diabetes, osteoporosis, etcetera, or you should proceed with caution, and be sure to talk to your doctor before you start any exercise activity.

Your Fitness Level: If you have been inactive for some time, rather than starting with one of the more strenuous exercises, **beginners of all ages should initially confine themselves to walking** until they can easily walk two miles at a brisk pace. When you reach this stage more strenuous exercises can be attempted if desired. Furthermore, some sports medicine physicians contend that **if you are badly overweight you should limit your exercise to walking** until you have lost weight to the point where you are less than 25 percent overweight.

Your Exercise Goals: If you want to strengthen your heart and lungs, improve your aerobic capacity and burn a lot of calories select an aerobic activity. If you want to improve your flexibility select a stretching type exercise. And if you want to become physically stronger choose one of the strength-building exercises.

Your Schedule: Only you know what the demands on your time from work, family and your social life are. What is the best time of day for you? Which days of the week best fit your schedule? Of course, you must be open to rearranging your priorities to fit exercise into your daily life.

Outdoors or Indoors: If you decide to exercise outdoors you should also have an alternate indoor activity, an activity you can fall back on in bad weather. For example, if you choose to jog outside early in the morning before work, you may want to purchase a treadmill for use at home on days when it is either too hot, too cold or the weather is bad.

Alone or with Others: On the plus side, an exercise partner can make exercise more enjoyable and can help you get going and keep going on days when you might otherwise quit. On the other hand, a partner probably means that you have the schedules of two people to contend with and plan around, which can at times actually hinder your workout.

How Much Are You Prepared to Spend: For many activities, you will need little or no special equipment. For instance, walking outside only requires comfortable shoes; whereas, joining and working out at a fitness center can be relatively expensive.

Aerobic (Cardio) Exercise

An aerobic exercise program should be vigorous enough to condition the cardiovascular system but not so strenuous as to exceed safe limits. Logically, how hard you should exercise is largely dependent on your age.

Some experts define safe as an exercise pace that is "comfortable." What they mean is that if, for instance, you are jogging or walking briskly you should be able to converse comfortably with a partner. They add that you should be breathing and feeling normally within ten minutes after you stop exercising – otherwise you are exercising too vigorously. Other signs that you are pushing too hard include difficulty breathing, feeling faint, or feeling weak – during or after exercising. If you experience any of these symptoms, you are exercising too intensely and you should cut back.

Other experts prefer a more quantitative definition. Two techniques used to judge how hard you should exercise during an endurance activity are the Target Heart Rate method (THR) and the Target Training Zone method (TTZ). For both methods, the objective is to raise your pulse through exercise to a specific range and hold it there for an extended period to obtain a cardiovascular benefit. This is the so-called heart-rated theory of exercise, which relies on heart rate (or pulse) to establish the proper exercise intensity.

Target-Heart Rate Method

The Target Heart Rate method (THR) is recommended by the American Heart Association. As shown in Table 10, the THR describes how fast the average person's heart should beat while performing an endurance exercise. For seniors who use THR, Table 10 presents an estimate of the THR you should gradually try to achieve. "Gradually" is the operative word. Going immediately from an inactive lifestyle to exercising at the Target Heart Rate range shown in the Table 10 can be dangerous and is not advised.

Age (years)	Max Average Heart Rate	Exercise Target Heart Rate*
50	170	85 to 128
55	165	83 to 124
60	160	80 to 120
65	155	78 to 116
70	150	75 to 113
75	145	73 to 109
80	140	70 to 105
* 50 to 75% of max heart rate		

Table 10: AHA Target Heart Rates

One way to reach your THR gradually is to take your pulse during

and endurance-type activity that is already a part of your life (while walking, for example.) Walk at your normal pace and record your heart rate over several sessions. Then over time, walk faster, so that your pulse rate gradually increases. Again over time, gradually try to get your heart rate up to 75 percent of the maximum rate shown in Table 10. **Never exceed the 75% of the maximum heart rate for your age**. Again, to be safe, check with your physician before starting an exercise program.

Target-Training Zone Method

The Target-Training Zone (TTZ) is a slightly different, and some say more reliable, measure of aerobic exercise intensity because it takes into account not only your age but also your resting pulse rate. Use the following procedure to calculate your target-training zone:

35

1) Calculate your **Maximum heart rate** = 220 minus your Age. (Your maximum heart rate is the fastest your heart can beat, and you definitely must exercise well below this level.)

2) Compute your **Maximum heart rate reserve** = Maximum heart rate − Resting pulse.

3) Lastly, calculate your **TTZ** pulse = (Maximum heart rate reserve multiplied by Exercise intensity level) + Resting pulse.

If you would rather not do the mathematics, use Table 11 to determine your TTZ. But before that, you need to determine the exercise intensity level that is right for you.

Intensity-Level Guidelines

Many exercise physiologists recommend that anyone over 50 years old, and especially seniors who are starting a physical fitness program after many years of inactivity, should begin exercising at 40 to 50% of their TTZ. Over time, gradually try to increase your exercise intensity level – but never exceed 75% of your TTZ.

Moderately active healthy seniors who, for example, have been walking at least two or three miles per day regularly can begin exercising at 50 to 65% of their TTZ. Again, over time, gradually try to increase your exercise intensity level – but again never exceed 75% of your TTZ.

If you do use the target-training zone approach, your pulse becomes your exercise guide. In addition, after a couple of months of aerobic exercise a sure indication that you are rounding into shape, making progress, is that your resting pulse slows down somewhat – especially if it was relatively fast at the start. This is because well-conditioned strengthened hearts are more efficient and so beat more slowly at rest.

Trained athletes often have a resting pulse of 50 beats per minute or lower, whereas the "average" pulse is 72 to 76 for untrained men and 75 to 80 for untrained women. Furthermore, as you become more physically fit you might have to exercise more vigorously to get your exercising pulse rate into your target-training zone.

When Not to Trust Your Pulse

The THR and TTZ methods, however, are not always the best way for older adults to decide how hard to exercise. This is because many seniors have long-standing medical conditions or take medications that change their heart rate. Instead, the **Borg scale** discussed in the next section may be a more

Age	Resting Pulse	Exercise Intensity (%)				
		40	50	60	70	80
50	60	104	115	126	137	148
	70	110	120	130	140	150
	80	116	125	134	143	152
55	60	102	113	123	134	144
	70	108	118	127	137	146
	80	114	123	131	140	148
60	60	100	110	120	130	140
	70	106	115	124	133	142
	80	112	120	128	136	144
65	60	98	108	117	127	136
	70	104	113	121	130	138
	80	110	118	125	133	140
70	60	96	105	114	123	132
	70	102	110	118	126	134
	80	108	115	122	129	136
75	60	94	103	111	120	128
	70	100	108	115	123	130
	80	106	113	119	126	132
80	60	92	100	108	116	124
	70	98	105	112	119	126
	80	104	110	116	122	128

Table 11: Target-Training Zone: 50 to 80

appropriate measure for seniors. Of course, some older exercisers who are in basically good health and who like a more "scientific approach" may find the THR or TTZ methods more to their liking. In any case all seniors should check with their doctor before embarking on any exercise program.

You definitely should not use the THR or TTZ approach if you take medications that change your heart rate, if you have a pacemaker for your heart, if you have an irregular heart rhythm, or if you have any other condition that affects your pulse rate. All of these situations can produce inaccurate pulse readings.

For example, many older adults take a class of medications called "beta blockers" for high blood pressure which lowers their heart rate. (Some eye drops used to treat glaucoma also contain beta blockers.) As discuss, your heart rate is a reflection of how hard your body is working.

But beta blockers tend to keep your heart rate slower, so no matter how hard you push yourself, you might never reach your target heart rate. You could easily overexert yourself, as you try in vain to reach a heart rate that the beta blocker you are taking won't allow. Being on beta blockers doesn't mean you can't exercise vigorously; it just means you can't rely on Table 10 or Table 11, or your pulse rate, to judge how hard you are working.

Again, all seniors should check with their doctor before embarking on any exercise program.

Listen to Your Body

Nobody can tell you how fast you should walk to reach a particular exercise intensity level, because an exercising level that is easy for one person might be strenuous for another. An alternative approach to the heart-rated theory of exercise is the "listen to your body" approach. Researchers have found that the level of effort you feel you put into an activity is likely to agree with the effort that actual physical measurements would reveal. In other words, if your body tells you that the exercise you are doing is moderate, your measured heart rate would probably show that it actually is working at a moderate level. (During moderate activity you can sense that you are challenging yourself but that you aren't near your limit.)

One way you can estimate how hard you should exercise is by using a measurement called the Borg scale, shown in Table 12 (on page 39). The Borg scale ranges from 6 (least effort) to 20 (maximum effort). For endurance activities, you should gradually work your way up to level 13 – the feeling that you are working at a somewhat hard level. Some people might feel that way when they are walking on flat ground; others might feel that way when they are jogging up a hill. Both are right. Remember, only you know how hard an exercise feels.

Level	Effort	Type of Training
6	Least effort	
7	Very, very light	
8		
9	Very light	
10		
11	Fairly light	Endurance
12		Endurance

38

13	Somewhat hard	Endurance
14		
15	Hard	Strength
16		Strength
17	Very Hard	Strength
18		
19	Very, very hard	
20		
	Maximum effort	

Table 12: Borg Scale for Exercise Intensity

Cardio: How Long & How Often?

The American College of Sports Medicine recommends that an exercise heart rate of 60 to 80 percent of your maximum heart rate should be maintained for about 30 to 45 minutes three to five days per week to become reasonably fit. They also stated, "For most people exercising at the lower end of their heart rate range for a longer time is better than exercising at the higher end of the range for a shorter time." The United States Surgeon General recommends that people accumulate 30 minutes of moderate activity on most, if not all, days of the week. More recently, the U.S. Institute of Medicine suggested 60 minutes of moderate exercise every day. To confuse matters even more, many exercise physiologists favor the following exercise schedule:

Low Exercise-Intensity Level (40 to 50% of maximum heart rate reserve): People in this category (particularly seniors – because of their age or lack of fitness) should work up to exercising 60 minutes per day at least five days per week. Despite the low intensity exercise level participants will attain what exercise physiologists feel is an acceptable – albeit minimum – level of fitness.

Moderate Exercise-Intensity Level (50 to 65% of maximum heart rate reserve): Seniors at this level should build up to 45 minutes of exercise per day at least five days per week to achieve a minimum fitness level.

High Exercise-Intensity Level (65 to 80% of maximum heart rate reserve): In this category, seniors need only exercise 30 minutes per day at least five days per week for a minimally acceptable fitness level.

As you can see, in general if you exercise at the lower exercise intensity levels your workout should last longer. Moreover, the longer and more frequently you exercise the greater your fitness reward. How fit you become is really a matter of your age, your genes, how fit you think you should be – and how hard you are willing to work. **But don't overdo it!** Again, it is worth repeating, every senior should have medical clearance before beginning any exercise program.

Pulse Measurement

In order to monitor the intensity of exercise, you should occasionally stop during your workout and take your pulse <u>immediately</u>. This is because your pulse will fall quickly once you stop exercising. The trick is to find your pulse within a couple of seconds and then start counting.

Quickly place the tips of two fingers on one of the two carotid arteries in your neck. (Your carotid arteries are located on either side of your throat.) Count the beats for ten seconds and multiply by six. For example, if you count 20 beats in ten seconds then your pulse would be 20x6 = 120 beats per minute.

You are doing fine if your pulse is within your TTZ range. If your pulse is too slow, exercise somewhat harder (if you can); if your pulse is fast, exercise easier. Again, after you have exercised for some time you will be able to feel that you are exerting the correct amount of effort and need only check your exercising pulse about once a week.

<u>Resting Pulse:</u> The best way to find your resting pulse is to take it immediately upon rising in the morning. Use the average over three days for the truest measure.

Aerobic Exercise: Typical Workout

First, do not smoke before you exercise (or after for that matter); do not eat for two hours before you start exercising, and refrain from drinking any alcohol for four hours prior to beginning your exercise routine. **A classic aerobic exercise routine consists of a warm up, your main exercise, and a cool down.**

1)   Start with a three to seven minute warm up. Three minutes of stretching is sufficient if you are going to engage in a low intensity exercise such as
badminton; whereas a longer seven-minute warm up is better preparation for a high intensity aerobic exercises such as jogging, cycling or stair climbing.

2) Then move on to 30 to 60 minutes of your main aerobic exercise.

3) Finish with a three to seven minute cool down period. Once more, if you are finishing a low-intensity exercise three minutes is enough. After a moderate or high-intensity aerobic exercise a seven minute cool down is more appropriate.

Warm up: Going from a resting state to a moderate or high-intensity exercise is a large jump. The warm up period gives your body time to bridge the gap and get ready for the more strenuous exercise that follows. Begin your warm up by walking slowly and gradually increase your pace as you approach the end of the warm up period. Next stretch. **Never stretch cold muscles.** Many stretches are based on yoga, where you start with good posture and then use your body weight to stretch your tissues. The following is a list of stretching exercises for your arms, neck, back and legs that are especially suited for warm up and cool down periods. Stretches (c) through (g) are illustrated in Figure 1 on page 42. (Some of these stretches can be done toward the end of the walking segment of your warm-up.) Perform the stretches as described.

a) Neck Swivel: From a standing position, with your arms hanging loosely, rotate your head about your neck, five times clockwise, then five times counter clockwise.

b) Shoulder Roll: While standing, with your arms hanging loosely at your side rotate your shoulders first in a forward motion, then backwards. Repeat five times.

c) Arm Pumping: Again, from a standing position, raise your elbows to shoulder height. Pull your elbows and arms slowly rearward as you thrust your chest forward. Repeat five times.

d) Side to side Stretch: From a standing position, raise both hands over your head. Bend slowly from side to side. Repeat five times.

e) Toe Touch: Sit along a bench and place your right leg on the bench. Position your left leg on the floor. Lean forward and try to touch your right toe until feel a stretch behind your right knee and calf. Do not bounce. Hold for a count of ten. Repeat with left leg raised. (This stretch can also be done from a standing position by placing a leg on a chair.)

f) Wall Push to Stretch Calves: Stand about two feet from a wall. Then as you extend your arms forward lean into the wall. Keep both heels flat on the floor. Do not bounce. Hold this position for a count of ten.

g) Quad Stretch: Balance yourself by placing your left hand on a wall. Bend your right leg and move your right heel toward your rear end. Grab your right foot with your right hand. Pull very gently. You should feel mild pressure in your right quad (the front of your right thigh). Do not bounce. Hold for a count of ten. Repeat for the left leg.

Do not feel limited to the preceding stretching exercises. There are many, many other good stretches available (too many to discuss here) that you might prefer.

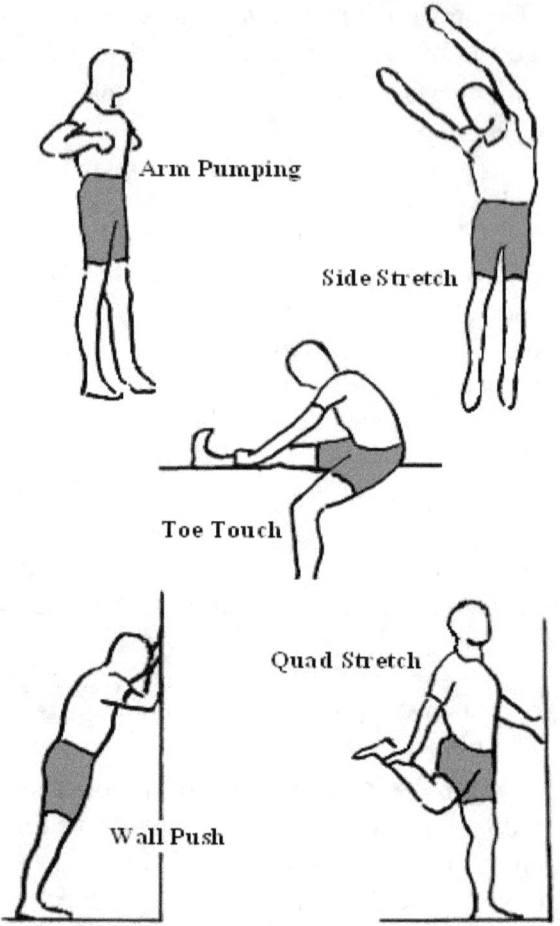

Figure 2: Stretching Exercises

    If your main activity is a low-intensity exercise, you can conclude your warm up after stretching out. If you are going on to a moderate or high-intensity aerobic exercise, after stretching start your main aerobic exercise but at a relatively lower level. Over the next few minutes gradually increase the intensity so that your pulse approaches your target training zone. For
instance, if you are a jogger you might warm up as follows: Start by walking slowly but steadily walk faster. After approximately five minutes stop and do two minutes of stretching. In theory, your warm up is over, but begin the main portion of your exercise by walking much faster, transition to a slow jog, then jog somewhat faster, and so on until, after about five minutes you have reached your regular jogging pace.

Main Exercise: Now you can begin your aerobic exercise of choice in earnest, stopping only to see that your pulse is in your target-training zone. If not, adjust your exercise level, exerting more or less effort. (Eventually, you will be able to sense that you are exercising at the correct intensity level and need only monitor your pulse occasionally.)

Cool Down: A five to seven-minute cooling off period should follow an aerobic workout. During cool down keep moving, decrease your activity level slowly. End your workout with leg stretches such as toe touches, a wall push and a quad stretch.

Walking Program

If your goal is to improve your general health and fitness, walking is a wonderful exercise. It's an exercise that you can do anywhere, that you can do outdoors or indoors, that requires no special equipment other than a good comfortable pair of walking shoes, and that you can do well into your old age. Walking does have a downside. Because it is a relatively low-intensity exercise, to get a good workout you have to spend more time walking compared to most high-intensity exercises.

Most seniors, especially those that have been sedentary for some time, are advised to start with a walking program that slowly but surely builds in intensity. If you walk hard enough, long enough and often enough, a walking workout can make you fit. A ten-week beginner's routine is shown in Table 13 (on page 44).

The first session in week 1 starts cautiously with approximately three minutes of warm-up walking at a very easy pace of about 4 kph. Continue your warm up with two minutes of stretching. (See the stretching exercises described earlier.) Then start walking more briskly, about 5.5 kph, but you should check your pulse and increase or decrease this to get your heart rate to a TTZ corresponding to about a 50 percent intensity level. After eight minutes, start your cool down by reducing your walking speed again to about 4 kph for three minutes. Conclude your session by doing about two minutes of stretching. The total workout time in week 1 is 18 minutes. The only part that changes in succeeding weeks (2 through 10), is the brisk walking portion of the workout increases continually from 8 minutes in week 1 to 30 minutes in week 10.

Week	Warm up (Minutes)		Brisk Walking (Minutes)	Cool down (Minutes)		Total Minutes
	Walk	Stretch		Walk	Stretch	
1	3	2	8	3	2	18
2	3	2	10	3	2	20
3	3	2	12	3	2	22
4	3	2	14	3	2	24
5	3	2	16	3	2	26
6	3	2	18	3	2	28
7	3	2	20	3	2	30
8	3	2	23	3	2	33
9	3	2	26	3	2	36
10	3	2	30	3	2	40

Table 13: Walking Program for Beginners

Walk at least three days a week for ten weeks. If you find a week particularly tiring, backup to the previous week, or repeat the week before continuing with the program. This is not a contest; you do not have to finish the program in ten weeks. Once you complete the ten-week program you can either stay on a walking routine, or go on to one of the more strenuous aerobic exercises.

If you decide to become a walker and want to improve, first go from walking three days per week to five days per week – at the same TTZ. To improve further gradually increase your total workout time from 40 to 60 minutes. To improve even more, gradually increase your walking speed, and TTZ, so that your exercise intensity level approaches 60 percent. Another way to increase the intensity of your walking workout is to include some hills in your route. Incidentally, as you would expect, walking over hilly terrain also burns more calories than walking on level ground. On the two days you don't walk, try to get in 20 minutes of strengthening exercises.

Because you will undoubtedly do most of your walking outside, you have to be aware of the weather forecast and have a backup plan for inclement weather. On bad-weather days, you could use an indoor walking site (like a mall, or an indoor track), walk on a treadmill, or do stretching or strength exercises instead of walking.

Get a Pedometer and Step Out

Sedentary people only take about 2000 to 3000 steps a day. For the average person with a stride equal to about 0.75 m, 2100 steps amounts to walking about one mile 1.6 km. A Harvard University study has shown that 6000 steps a day correlate with lower death rates in men, and that 8000 to 10000 step per day promote weight loss. And these health and weight management benefits don't oblige you to walk continuously until you accrue the required number of steps. Rather, all steps throughout the day to wherever and whenever count toward your daily total. (Some pedometers also show total "aerobic steps," correctly defined as those steps accumulated during at least 10 minutes of continuous walking at a rate of at least 60 steps per minute.) Because 10000 steps a day may not be achievable by some people, particularly by those who are elderly, sedentary, or who have chronic diseases, rather than insisting on a blanket 10000 steps per day, a stepping goal should be based on an individual's baseline steps plus an increment of additional steps. (Your baseline is the number of steps taken in an average day.)

A pedometer (or an App on your Smart Phone) can keep track of your steps. And a study by the American College of Sports Medicine found that participants who used pedometers were motivated to add about 2000 steps to their daily routine. To start a stepping program, buy a pedometer. Wear the pedometer for a week and determine the number of steps you take on an average day. This is your baseline. Then add the equivalent of half an hour of walking to your day, or roughly 2500 extra steps per day. For example, consider a woman who wears a pedometer and notes that on an average day she accumulates 3500 steps. Her goal should be to add the equivalent of a half hour of walking to her day, or roughly 2500 more steps per day, for a daily total of 6000 steps.

There are many little ways to add steps to your day, such as taking stairs rather than an elevator, parking further from your destination, pacing as you talk on the telephone, marching-in-place for a minute once every hour – and of course taking short walks whenever you can. So buy a pedometer – get off the couch and step out for your health!

Jogging Program

If you are a younger senior in good condition, have completed the "Walking Program for Beginners," or have been walking regularly, and have medical clearance, you may want to start a jogging program. Table 14 illustrates a 13-week beginner's schedule. Try to get your pulse into your TTZ but don't overdue it. Gradually, over time, you want to increase both the intensity and distance of your jogging routine. However, if you don't have the physical makeup to do both, always choose endurance over intensity; i.e., choose distance rather than speed, choose to jog longer rather than faster.

Week	Warm up (Minutes)		Brisk Walking & Jogging (Minutes)	Cool down (Minutes)		Total Minutes
	Walk	Stretch		Walk	Stretch	
1	5	2	Walk 5 Jog 3 Walk 5 Jog 3	3	2	28
2	5	2	Walk 4 Jog 5 Walk 4 Jog 5	3	2	30
3	5	2	Walk 4 Jog 5 Walk 4 Jog 5	3	2	30
4	5	2	Walk 4 Jog 6 Walk 4 Jog 6	3	2	32
5	5	2	Walk 4 Jog 7 Walk 4 Jog 7	3	2	34
6	5	2	Walk 4 Jog 8 Walk 4 Jog 8	3	2	36
7	5	2	Walk 4 Jog 9 Walk 4 Jog 9	3	2	38
8	5	2	Walk 4 Jog 12	3	2	28
9	5	2	Walk 4 Jog 15	3	2	31
10	5	2	Walk 4 Jog 17	3	2	33
11	5	2	Walk 2 Slow Jog 2 then Jog 17	3	2	33
12	5	2	Walk 2 Slow Jog 4 then Jog 17	3	2	35
13	5	2	Slow Jog 6 then Jog 17	3	2	35

Table 14: Jogging Program for Beginners

Jog at least three days a week for 13 weeks. Again, if you find a week particularly tiring, backup to the previous week, or repeat the week before continuing with the program. Once you complete the program, if you want to improve, first go from jogging three days per week to five days per week – at the same TTZ. To improve further gradually increase your total workout time from 30 to 60 minutes. To improve even more, gradually increase your jogging speed, and TTZ, so that your exercise intensity level approaches 65 percent. Another good way to increase the intensity of your jogging workout is to try to include some hills in your workout. On the two days you don't walk, try to get in 20 minutes of strengthening exercises.

Because you will undoubtedly do most of your jogging outside, you have to be aware of the weather forecast and have a contingency plan for inclement weather. On bad-weather days, you might use an indoor track, try an alternate exercise like jogging on a treadmill, or do stretching or strength exercises.

As always, stop exercising immediately if you experience tightness or pain in your chest, become lightheaded or dizzy, are severely breathless, lose muscle control or are nauseous. These are warning signs of over-exertion and you definitely should lower your exercise-intensity level. If you experience these symptoms, it is also a good idea to seek medical attention.

Be aware that the pounding your body gets from jogging usually takes its toll over time. Many joggers have recurring, nagging injuries, particularly to their legs and feet. If you begin to suffer chronic injuries, remember there are other high-intensity aerobic exercises for which your body might be better suited. At that point, you might consider switching to cycling, a rowing machine.

Strength-Building Programs

As good as aerobic exercises are, they contribute little to building upper-body strength. And strength training can increase your muscle mass, which tends to increase your basal metabolic rate – and helps you control your weight.

If you are a beginner interested in strength training it's probably worthwhile to start by joining a health club, where you can get professional instruction on the proper use of exercise equipment, from dumbbells to rowing machines, and where you can compare different exercise routines. Another possibility is to hire a personal trainer for a couple of sessions to get you started on a program personalized to your fitness level and to teach you correct exercise techniques.

Dumbbell Exercises

Of all the many strength-building options, I personally prefer free weights (actually dumbbells) because they can be used at home. Working out at home has some significant advantages. First, your workout takes less time because you don't have to drive back and forth to a fitness facility; second, you have the flexibility of dividing your workout into small time segments to fit your day, whenever you have time, such as when the baby is napping, and of course working out at home is certainly less expensive.

You can workout in a bedroom, basement, garage, attic – anywhere you have extra space. A set of variable (adjustable) weight dumbbells and a small weight bench don't take up much room and are all you need for a home-based gym. (Bear in mind, **knowledge and the discipline to work out regularly are far more important than fancy equipment**.) Before investing in a set of weights and a bench, however, it may still be worthwhile to start by joining a health club. At a health club you can get expert instruction on the use of free weights. And you may find that you actually prefer to workout at a club.

But if you do decide to opt for the convenience of a home-based gym, that would be the time to purchase a pair of variable-weight dumbbells and a strong weight bench (that will not tip over) for home use. Rather than an entire set of weights, purchase just enough dumbbell weight so that you can do a military press five times.

If you are 50, 60, 70, or more, you should adjust the types of exercises, number of sets and repetitions and the intensity of your workout. The seven dumbbell exercises that follow comprise a total-body workout, suitable for seniors and beginners of all ages, that involve every major muscle group. (Regardless of age the mechanics of dumbbell training are the same.) When done consecutively without stopping a series of exercises is called a circuit. To start, use the same dumbbell weight for all the exercises, a weight that allows you to do 10 to 15 repetitions of the most difficult exercise in the circuit. For the first week do one circuit per training session.

Your goal should be two circuits per session, which should take you about 20 minutes (with a two to three-minute rest between circuits). When you are comfortable at this level you are ready to increase the dumbbell weight – but by no more than roughly 10 percent (or ½ kg minimum). The seven exercises are illustrated in Figures 2 and 3 (on pages 50 and 51). Perform about 10 repetitions of each exercise.

a) **Bench Press**: With your head and back on the bench, hold a dumbbell in each hand to the side of your shoulders, palms facing each other. Slowly raise the dumbbells extending your arms above your shoulders. Pause, then lower the dumbbells down to the starting position. The bench press primarily works your pectorals, triceps and deltoids.

b) **One–Arm Dumbbell Row**: Hold a dumbbell in your right hand, palm facing toward your right thigh. Stand to the right of your weight bench and place your left knee on the bench. Support yourself by putting your left hand on the bench. (Flex your right knee slightly and lean forward so your back is almost parallel to the floor.) Slowly pull your right arm up until your upper arm is parallel to the floor. (Keep your right arm close to your torso.) Pause and lower your right arm to the starting position. After you complete a set, stand to the left of the bench and repeat the exercise with the dumbbell in your left hand. Rows mainly work your latissimus dorsi and rhomboid muscles.

c) **Seated Shoulder Press**: From a seated position, hold a dumbbell in each hand to the side of your shoulders, palms facing forward. Slowly raise the weights over your head until your arms are straight. Pause, then lower the
dumbbells to the starting position. The shoulder press mainly exercises your deltoids, trapezius, triceps, latissimus dorsi and rhomboid muscles.

d) **Curls for Biceps**: Stand with a dumbbell in each hand, your arms hanging loosely, with your palms to the side your thighs and facing straight ahead. Keep your elbows tucked into your side and slowly lift the dumbbells until they are approximately shoulder high. Pause and lower the dumbbells to the starting position. Curls chiefly work your biceps.

e) **Tricep Extension**: With a dumbbell in your right hand, assume the same initial position as in the one-arm dumbbell row. Slowly move your right arm rearward until it is nearly parallel to the floor. Pause and then return the dumbbell to the starting position without bending your arm. After completing a set, stand to the left of the bench and repeat the exercise with the dumbbell in your left hand. This exercise mainly works your triceps.

f) **Front Squats**: Stand with a dumbbell in each hand, to the side of your shoulders, palms facing each other (inward). Slowly bend your knees and lower your body until your thighs are almost parallel to the floor. Try to keep your heels on the floor. Pause and gradually raise your body by straightening your knees. Squats work your gluteus, quadriceps and hamstrings.

g) **Curls for Abs**: This is not a weight lifting exercise but is a useful part of any routine. Lie face up on a floor mat with your hands folded over your chest and your legs bent. Keeping your feet flat on the mat, slowly curl your torso up and toward your thighs until your shoulder blades are off the mat. Pause, then return to the starting position. This exercise works your rectus abdominis muscles – your abs.

Remember to do about five minutes of aerobic and stretching exercises before and after your strength exercises, and to workout two to three (non-consecutive) days per week. Why non-consecutive days? Because strengthening exercises work a muscle until it's fatigued, and a day off is needed for muscles to recover, repair and rebuild. And listen to your body to determine your level of exertion. Don't over do it!

A final word about breathing properly: Never hold your breath during weight training. This can cause your blood pressure to get dangerously high. Rather, breathe naturally and try to exhale during a lift.

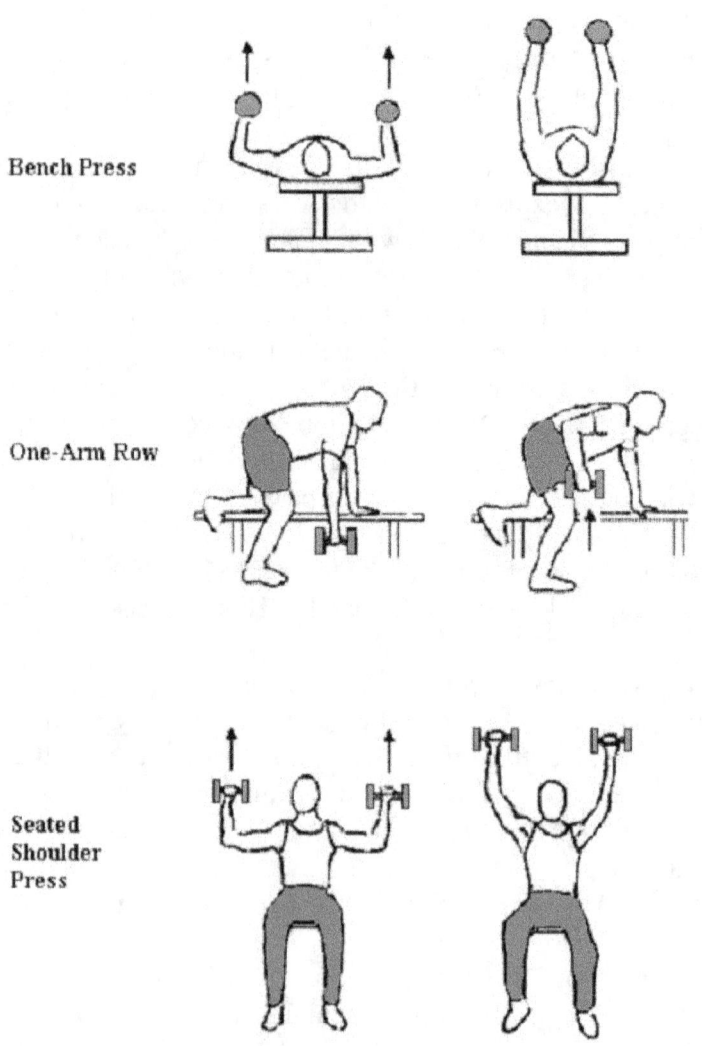

Bench Press

One-Arm Row

Seated Shoulder Press

Figure 3: Strengthening Exercises (a to c)

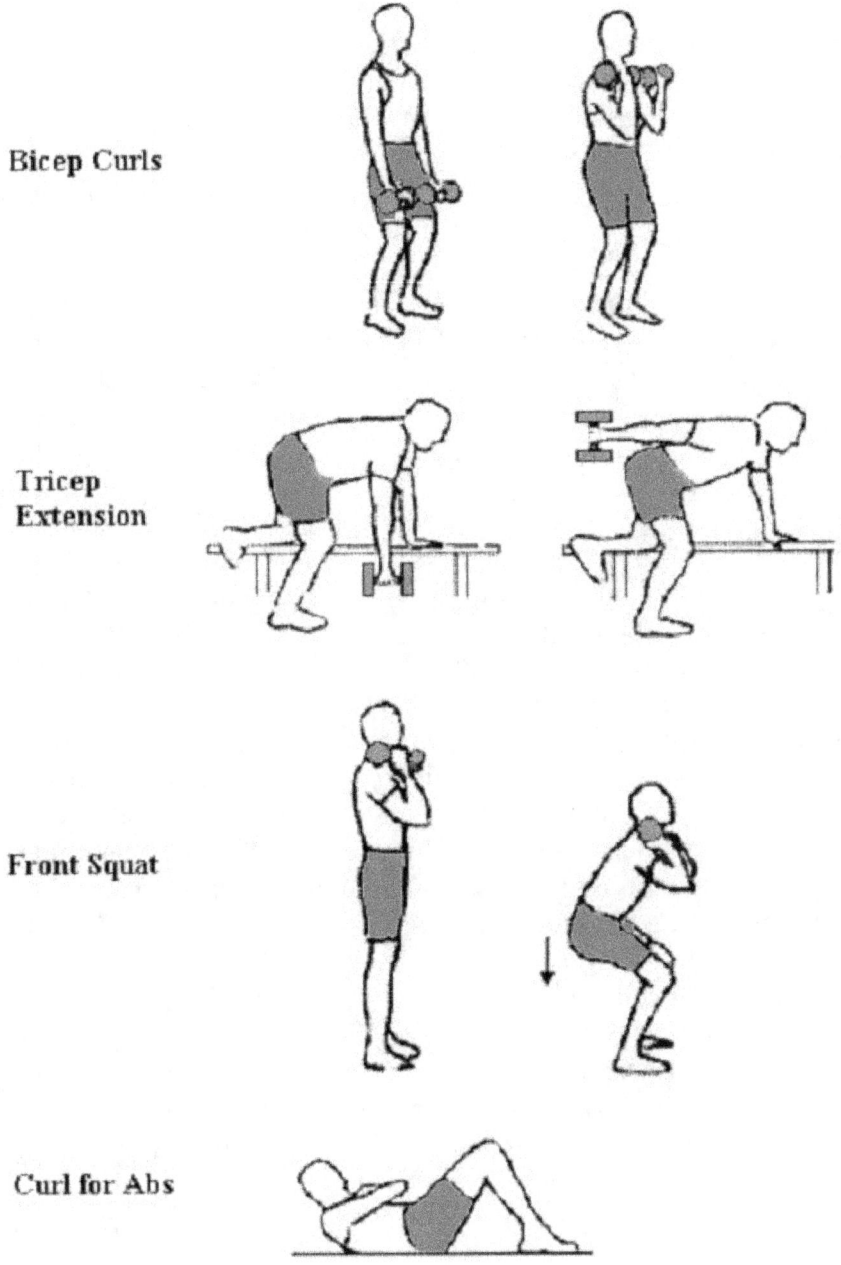

Bicep Curls

Tricep Extension

Front Squat

Curl for Abs

Figure 4: Strengthening Exercises (d to g)

Other Exercises

There are literally hundreds of other aerobic, flexibility and strengthening exercises. Too many to review here, but many are definitely worth considering. For instance, swimming laps in a pool provides an excellent low-impact aerobic workout that also builds strength. Of course, the disadvantage is that you need to join a fitness facility that has a pool. Some trainers think a good rowing machine provides a great total-body workout. Others feel a workout on a stairclimber is hard to beat. All have advantages and disadvantages.

In fact, most trainers recommend that you modify your routine every few months to add variety. Some advocate alternating exercises every other session. For instance, if you jog and lift weights on alternate days, you avoid repeating movements on consecutive days. As bonus, you will also most likely avoid the injuries that are often associated with day-after-day repetitive motion.

Missed Workouts

Inevitably, you will miss some aerobic or strengthening workouts. It may be because you're traveling, or due to a minor illness, or an injury. If you are ill or injured, wait for the injury to heal, or until you feel like your normal self before resuming your exercise routine. If you only miss a day or two, you can undoubtedly just pick up where you left off as if nothing happened. If you miss a week or more, however, you will probably have lost some of your fitness gains and might have to resume at a somewhat lower exercising-intensity level. This means that when you come back after missing some aerobic sessions, you might have to exercise at a slightly lower TTZ, or shorten the duration of your workout. And when you return after missing some strengthening sessions, you might want to reduce the weight you are lifting or reduce the number of repetitions.

Incidentally, physical fitness can be maintained only by regular workouts. If your exercise frequency drops to one day a week, half your fitness gains will be lost in 10 weeks. If exercise is stopped completely, virtually all your accumulated fitness benefits will be lost in five weeks! Therefore, if you want to keep that state of well-being, feeling better, looking better, it's important to make regular exercise part of your lifestyle.

Exercising in Hot Weather

When you engage in vigorous exercise, your body generates a great deal of heat, and your body temperature can rise from 37°C up to 38.5°C. (A body temperature of 40.5°C is life threatening.) High ambient temperatures and high humidity are a concern because both influence how effectively you transfer the heat your body generates to the environment. High ambient temperatures are an obvious cooling problem, but high levels of humidity also cause cooling difficulties by hindering the evaporation of perspiration. As a result, on days when it is both hot and humid it is even more difficult to transfer heat from your body to the surrounding ambient air. This combination can cause your body temperature to rise to dangerous levels. **On hot humid summer days, therefore, you must guard against overdoing it.**

Heat Index: Adopted by the U.S. National Weather Service, the heat index, or apparent temperature, combines the effects of air (dry bulb) temperature and relative humidity. (Heat index values are expressed in either degrees Fahrenheit or Celsius.) The heat index is not perfect but it is the best guide for the general population. As expected, Table 15 shows that when the heat index rises, so do health risks. In hot weather, the major health threats are heat stroke, heat exhaustion and dehydration.

Category	Heat Index (°F)	Heat-Related Risks
Caution	27 to 32°C	Unexpected fatigue possible with prolonged exposure and/or physical activity.
Extreme Caution	32 to 41°C	Muscle cramps and/or heat exhaustion possible with prolonged exposure and/or physical activity.
Danger	41 to 54°C	Muscle cramps and/or heat exhaustion likely. Heat stroke possible with long exposure and/or physical activity.
Extreme Danger	54°C or higher	Heat stroke likely.

Table 15: Health Risks in Hot Weather

Heat Exhaustion: When heat index values reach 32 to 41°C, you could suffer muscle cramps, particularly in your legs and heat exhaustion. The symptoms of heat exhaustion are pale clammy skin, dizziness or fainting, a rapid pulse, fast breathing, and nausea. If you experience any of these problems, get to a cool place, lie down and sip water. You may also need to seek medical attention.

Heat Stroke: Much more dangerous is heat stroke, which results when extremely hot weather triggers a malfunction of the body's thermostat, causing the body temperature to rise to 40°C or higher. Symptoms of heat stroke are confusion or loss of consciousness, flushed, hot and dry skin, a strong and rapid pulse. **Heat stroke is a medical emergency**. Move the person to the coolest accessible place and call local emergency phone number. Some first aid measures include removing some of the person's clothing and sponging with cool water.

Dehydration: Everyone knows drinking water is important for good health, but it's even more important on hot days while you are exercising. During vigorous exercise, you can lose one to two quarts of water per hour in sweat, so it's essential to use common sense and stay hydrated. And in hot weather, drink plenty of water and fruit juice even if you don't feel thirsty.

Exercising in Cold Weather

The ideal exercise temperature range is about 4 to 29°C with a wind speed less than 25 kph, but many people continue to exercise outdoors at temperatures well below 4°C. Generally, cold weather is less dangerous to an exerciser – but definitely not risk-free. When you exercise outdoors in cold weather you encounter an entirely new set of difficulties. Besides often- treacherous footing on snow-covered or icy surfaces, you must contend with low temperatures and the wind.

Wind Chill Temperature Index: Basic physics states that when heat leaves an object the temperature of the object drops. The same principle applies to your body. As heat leaves your body, your temperature drops and you feel cold. Very low ambient temperatures combined with the wind increase the amount of heat leaving your body. As the wind speed increases, the temperature of any exposed skin drops even further. The Wind Chill Temperature Index was developed in an effort to quantify this phenomenon, and is a measure of the relative discomfort due to combined cold temperature and wind. In essence, the wind-chill temperature lets you know what the outside air temperature "feels like," based on the heat loss from skin exposed to low air temperatures and the wind.

One of the **potential consequences of very low wind-chill temperatures is frostbite**. Table 16 (on the next page) employs the Canadian interpretation of frostbite risks rather than the U.S. version.

(After all, who knows more about cold weather than Canadians?) **Other serious cold weather related conditions are hypothermia and heart attack.**

Frostbite: When body tissue freezes the injury is called frostbite, which usually strikes fingers, toes, nose and ears. Frostbitten skin is numb, hard and pale, and requires immediate medical attention. If you suspect you have frostbite, get indoors as quickly as you can and call or send for help. First aid steps include covering the frozen area with a blanket and drinking a warm nonalcoholic beverage.

Wind Chill Temperature	Frostbite Risk	Exposure Minutes
4°C to -27°C	Low	---
-28°C to -37°C	Medium	10 to 30
-37°C to -47°C	High	5 to 10
-48°C to -53°C	Higher	2 to 5
-54°C to -67°C	Highest	2 or less

Table 16: Frostbite Risk vs. Wind-Chill

Hypothermia: Prolonged exposure to extreme cold, especially during exercise, can result in a depletion of energy stores (calories) which can cause a drop in body temperature. This in turn can cause gradual mental slowing. The stricken person becomes increasingly unreasonable, clumsy, irritable, sleepy, and eventually lapses into a coma. This is a life-threatening condition. Severe hypothermia can lead to cardiac and respiratory failure and death. To help, your first move should be to call your local emergency number. Then start first aid (which is beyond the scope of this book).

Heart Attack: As the air temperature drops, your body's air-warming system may not be able to adequately heat the cold air entering your mouth and flowing down your windpipe. As a result, the incoming cold air may cause your coronary arteries to constrict – resulting in a heart attack – particularly if you are not in good condition.

Upshot of Cold Weather: Once the wind-chill temperature reaches about -12°C exercising outdoors becomes increasingly uncomfortable. Even if you are an outdoor enthusiast, **at -12°C wind chill and lower most seniors should switch to an indoor exercise venue** until the weather moderates. Join a health club, or set up a small workout space in your home, or walk in an enclosed mall.

Exercise Risks and Problems

Certain situations may occur that indicate you may be doing too much, exercising too hard. A feeling of having worked hard is fine, sweating is good, but not a feeling of undo fatigue.

Perhaps the most frequent problems faced by exercisers are injuries of the joints and muscles: sprains and strains, knee pain, elbow pain, back pain, neck pain, shin splints and stress fractures. Most happen when you exercise too hard.

Potentially serious problems are signaled if you experience any of the following symptoms during or after exercise. The symptoms include but are not limited to any abnormal heart action such as an irregular heart rhythm; pain or pressure in the middle of your chest; pain in an arm or your neck; dizziness, fainting or lightheadedness; severe exhaustion; sudden loss of coordination; or confusion. If any of these symptoms are experienced, stop exercising immediately and get medical help.

Avoiding Injury

When he practiced, my retired friend and workout buddy, Dr. Kanaar's specialty was rehabilitation medicine but he also preached what he called "preventive medicine," that is avoiding injury by practicing a common-sense approach to exercise:

1) Have a medical checkup and then set realistic fitness goals.

2) Build up your exercise intensity gradually over many weeks, months.

3) After you eat a meal, wait two hours before exercising.

4) Buy good suitable clothing for your exercise routine.

5) Use safety and protective equipment when appropriate, such as helmet when you bicycle, and goggles when you play handball, squash or racquetball.

6) On hot days, follow the precautions in the section "Exercising in Hot Weather."

7) On cold days, follow the precautions in the section "Exercising in Cold Weather."

8) If you insist on working out in very hot or cold weather, always let someone know when and where you will be exercising and when you are planning to return.

9) If you are new to a gym or health club, attend an orientation session before you use any unfamiliar exercise equipment. Otherwise, read the operating instructions carefully and ask someone qualified to help you.

10) For aerobic activities, warm up slowly to reach your TTZ and cool down slowly after you exercise.

11) Do not increase the difficulty of any activity (e.g., your walking or jogging distance, the amount of weight you lift) by more than 10 percent per week.

12) Jog on softer surfaces such as a level grass field, a dirt path, or a running track.

13) After exercising wait 30 minutes before eating.

14) As a final point, if you experience some early warning pain stop exercising.

Minor Leg Injures: Many minor leg injuries can be treated using the well-known **R.I.C.E**. method, i.e., rest, ice, compression, elevation.

- Rest. You may not have to avoid all physical activity; just taking it easy might be fine.

- Ice. Apply ice for 15 minutes several times a day for as long as there is any swelling.

- Compress the area with a bandage or sleeve to help control swelling

- Elevate the injured area above the level of your heart.

My Exercise Routine

I started jogging in the late 1960's. Of course I was much younger then. I jogged three to five miles almost every morning and worked out with free weights (dumbbells) on the days I didn't jog. After 20 years of jogging, the constant pounding resulted in a troubling number of chronic minor leg and foot injuries. So I switched to walking and I have been walking ever since. Now I'm a semi-retired senior citizen. I have more time. For the past 20 years, from 6:00 to 7:00 am, I take a brisk walk covering slightly less than four miles. Most days I walk outside but when the weather is bad I head for a nearby shopping mall. For variety, some days I power walk in place for about 45 minutes using an exercise DVDs to set a rhythm; then I complete my workout doing two circuits of the dumbbell exercises described earlier.

In warmer weather I golf (walking 9 or 18 holes) or hike (about eight miles) two or three times a week. When I'm not golfing or hiking I go on my early morning walk. When I golf or hike – that's my workout. Although recently after I finished my brisk one-hour morning walk followed by 20 minutes of dumbbell exercises, a friend called later in the day and next thing I know I'm playing 18 holes of golf – walking of course. In total, I exercised 5 hours and 45 minutes, burned about 2000 kcalories, and felt strong, definitely not tired, at the end of the day. Not bad for a 75 year-old senior!

In summary, one day I walk outside for an hour; the following day I power walk in place for 40 minutes using an exercise DVD and also lift weights; the next day I'm back to walking outside again; and so on. I've been doing this for 15 years. I exercise every day without fail. Every day! My exercise routine combined with a sensible diet have kept me trim over the years (within three pounds of my college-graduation weight). Most people think I'm much younger than my chronological age – and I feel great!

Workout - Feel Good Stay Healthy

If your goal is a chiseled body with washboard abs and the endurance and strength of a triathlon athlete, you're reading the wrong book . Sure the aerobic and strength routines outlined here will help you get in shape, slim down and get somewhat stronger – but your body is not going to be transformed into the physique of a young world-class athlete.

This book is about how you should workout to get fit so that you feel good and stay healthy. And you're not going to get fit just because you join a fancy health club with lots of high-tech equipment – if you only workout once or twice a week, or every other week. Joining a health club is great – if you use it consistently.

The words that describe our kind of workout are consistent, determined, steady, persistent, dogged, unswerving, gritty, single-minded. Get the point? In our kind of workout, you decide that you will workout at least five days a week; that an aerobic exercise will form the core of your workout, and that you will incorporate some strengthening exercises two days a week.

After that, it doesn't matter exactly what exercises you choose, what equipment you use, or what facility you use. These are secondary factors. What matters most is that you exercise consistently. **To improve muscle tone and overall fitness, feel good and stay healthy, you should exercise at least five days per week, day after day, week after week, year after year – for as long as you are physically able.** Remember the key words: consistent, determined, steady, persistent, dogged, unswerving, gritty, single-minded. Consistent!

Of course, there's a bit more involved. To feel good and stay healthy, you must also eat properly. That's next in **NUTRITION for SENIORS**.

NUTRITION FOR SENIORS

Healthy eating habits, the result of sensible nutritional practices, must be an integral part of any physical fitness program. In this section you will learn how to improve the "nutritional quality" of the food you eat, and, as expected, we will also point out foods that you should avoid, i.e., those foods that are loaded with "nutritionally-empty calories."

Food is far more than just an energy source. Foods are made up of seven basic constituents: carbohydrates, proteins, fats, vitamins, minerals, fiber and water. (Some nutritionists would add phytochemicals to this list – but more on this later.) For a healthy body you need to eat the correct quantity and proportion of all these components. You need protein, carbohydrates and fats, for growth, repair and energy. You need vitamins and minerals, albeit in relatively small quantities, so they can perform their vital roles in the thousands of biochemical reactions in your body. Fiber, the broad name given to the stuff you eat that your body cannot digest, is needed to assist your digestive system.

Fortunately, supermarkets have all the foods we need – and in abundance. Yet most nutritionists agree that a great many Americans are not eating well enough to sustain good health. In general, our diet is too high in fat – with an average of 40 percent of our calories from fat – contributing to atherosclerosis. Another culprit is sugar. As a nation we consume more than 100 pounds of sugar per year per person, totaling an unhealthy, nutritionally empty, 500 kcalories per day. This large intake of sugar leads to obvious ills, such as obesity and tooth decay.

Add to this the increased use of processed and convenience foods, the proliferation of nutritional misinformation and deceptive advertising, and it is clear that most people must improve their understanding of nutrition in order to eat properly.

Nutrients & Micronutrients

Before we begin let us define some terms. Nutrients and micronutrients are the components of foods that are essential to human life. Proteins, carbohydrates and fats are nutrients. Some nutritionists refer to proteins, carbohydrates and fats as "macronutrients," and call vitamins and minerals "micronutrients" because they are present in foods in much smaller amounts than macronutrients.

More recently, a new grouping of naturally occurring plant-based chemicals, called phytochemicals, or phytonutrients by some nutritionists, have been identified as having many healthful qualities, but unlike traditional macronutrients and micronutrients, phytonutrients are not needed by humans to live; i.e., their absence will not necessarily result in metabolic problems, or in a deficiency disease.

Proteins are Building Blocks

Proteins are molecules of amino acids that are required for cell maintenance and repair, as well as for the regulation of a wide range of bodily functions. Humans need 22 amino acids in order to live. Our bodies can make 14 of the amino acids on their own, but eight of them, named the essential-amino acids, must be acquired from the foods we eat.

Some foods have all the amino acids needed to build other proteins. These are called complete proteins. Nearly every animal food, including dairy products, eggs, meat, poultry and fish are complete proteins because they contain all eight-essential amino acids. **Soy is the only plant-based food that has all eight essential-amino acids.**

Other plant-based protein sources lack one or more essential amino acids (i.e., amino acids that the body can neither create nor manufacture by modifying other amino acids.) These incomplete proteins are found in legumes, grains, nuts, and seeds. However, consuming combinations of foods that have incomplete proteins can provide the same complete protein end effect as animal protein. For a complete-protein meal, simply eat any of the incomplete plant proteins with another but different incomplete plant protein. Examples of some healthy plant-protein combinations that result in complete proteins are:

Eating grains with legumes: pasta & beans, rice & lentils, tortillas with refried beans, etc

Eating grains with nuts or seeds: such as peanut butter on whole-grain bread, etc

Around the world, millions of people do not get enough protein. Protein malnutrition can cause growth failure, loss of muscle mass, decreased immunity, weakening of the heart and respiratory system, and in some cases death. Whereas, in most developed countries, getting the minimum daily requirement of protein is usually not a problem, because almost any reasonable diet will provide most of us with sufficient protein.

Adults need about 0.79 grams of protein for every kilogram of body weight per day to keep from slowly breaking down their own tissue. A case in point, an adult weighing 70 kg requires about (70 x 0.70), or 55 grams of protein per day. How much protein is in food? A few examples: There are approximately seven grams of protein in 30 grams of beef, poultry, fish, cheese or peanuts. Soybeans pack 10 grams of protein per 30 grams. Most other beans and lentils contain about six grams of protein per 30 grams. There are roughly three grams of protein in 30 grams of whole-grain cereal, and milk has one gram of protein per 30 mL.

Understand that foods are rarely straight protein. Some high-protein foods, such as marbled beef and whole milk, also come with lots of unhealthy saturated fat. Therefore, when you eat meat, eat the leanest cuts, and when you consume dairy products, choose skim or low-fat varieties. On the other hand, beans, nuts, and whole grains offer high-quality (albeit incomplete) protein with little saturated fat – but with lots of healthful fiber and micronutrients.

You Need Carbs

Carbohydrates provide your body with its basic fuel, the energy your cells need to survive. The staple of most diets around the world, carbohydrates provide essential vitamins and minerals, fiber, and numerous beneficial compounds (phytonutrients) that promote good health.

The simplest carbohydrate is glucose. Glucose, also called "blood sugar" and "dextrose," flows in the bloodstream so that it is available to every cell in your body. Your body's cells absorb glucose and convert it into energy to drive the cell. Glucose is a simple sugar, meaning that it tastes sweet. Some other simple sugars are sucrose, also known as "white sugar," fructose, the main sugar in fruits, and lactose, the sugar found in milk. They all taste sweet, and most are digested and enter your bloodstream quickly. When you eat fruit or drink milk, however, the natural sugar comes with vitamins, minerals (and fiber in the case of fruit); whereas the simple sugars in candy, for instance, are nothing but nutritionally-empty calories.

Then there are the more complex carbohydrates. Most grains (wheat, corn, oats, rice) and foods like potatoes, pasta and plantains are complex carbohydrates. In general, but not always, complex carbohydrates are digested more slowly than simple carbohydrates, and take much longer to enter your bloodstream. Most of us have heard that eating complex carbohydrates is good, and eating sugar-loaded foods is a bad. The reason is that simple sugars require little digestion, and when you eat a sweet food, such as a candy bar, or drink a can of soda, your blood glucose level rises rapidly. In response, your pancreas secretes a large amount of insulin to keep your blood glucose levels from rising too high. The large insulin response in turn tends to cause your blood sugar to fall to levels that are too low. As a consequence, about three to five hours after consuming sweets you feel lethargic and hungry. Many people react to this by eating yet another sweet, which can start a rollercoaster ride of surging glucose and then insulin. None of this is experienced after eating most complex carbohydrates, or a balanced meal, because the digestion and absorption processes are much slower.

Glycemic Index

Thinking of carbohydrates as complex or simple, as good or bad, is outdated. More recently, a system has been devised to classify carbohydrates. The system, called the glycemic index (GI), measures the effect a carbohydrate has on your blood sugar - quantifying how rapidly and to what level your blood sugar rises after you eat a food containing carbohydrates, compared to a reference food (usually glucose or white bread). For instance, a candy bar, which is digested rapidly has a high GI and causes an almost immediate jump in your blood sugar; whereas, lentil soup is digested more slowly and has a low GI. The factors that influence a food's GI are:

Fiber prevents the rapid digestion of the carbohydrates in food and slows the discharge of sugar into the blood stream. Higher fiber content results in a lower GI.

Coarsely-ground grains are digested more slowly and have lower GI values than finely-ground grains.

Less-processed carbohydrates, such whole-grain foods where the fiber, bran and germ are intact, are digested more slowly than highly-processed carbohydrates. It follows, therefore, that less processing usually results in a lower GI.

Unripe fruits and vegetables contain less sugar and have a lower GI than ripe varieties.

More acid or fat a food has, the slower its carbohydrates are digested and absorbed into the blood stream. More acid and fat in a food mean a lower GI.

The glycemic index uses a scale of 0 to 100, with foods that cause the most rapid rise in blood sugar having the highest values. In this book and many others, glucose is the arbitrary reference food, and is assigned a GI = 100. (For a given food, a GI less than 56 is considered low, a GI = 56 to 69 is medium, and a GI greater than 69 is high.) Note that foods that contain little or no carbohydrate (such as meat, fish, eggs, avocado, wine, beer and other alcoholic beverages) do not have GI values.

Glycemic Load

Some food scientists have come to recognize that a food's GI value alone does not provide enough information to judge how a particular food will affect your blood sugar. This is because the GI does not take into account how much carbohydrate is in a food serving, and your blood sugar level is influenced by both the quality of the carbohydrate (GI) and the quantity of carbohydrate you eat. With this in mind, researchers developed a new guideline called the glycemic load (GL) which takes into account both a food's GI and the quantity of carbohydrate the food contains. A food's GL is calculated by multiplying the food's GI by the number of carbohydrate grams in a serving. For a given food, a **GL less 11 is considered low, a GL = 11 to 19 medium, and a GL greater than 19 is high**. Most people consume 60 to 180 GL units per day, with a GL of about 100 for a typical diet.

Table 17 (on page 64) shows the GI and GL values for some common foods. Most of the data are from the on-line database of the University of Sidney (Australia). The difference between a food's GI and GL is illustrated by a simple example. Table 17 indicates watermelon has a GI = 72, quite high. In this case, however, GI alone is misleading because watermelon only has about six grams of carbohydrate per serving. (Watermelon is almost entirely water, with some fiber and a small quantity of carbohydrate.) So a typical serving of watermelon, has a GL = GI x (net carb grams) = 0.72 x 6 = 4.3, which is quite low. (Note in the calculation, watermelon's GI value has been converted from 72% to the decimal equivalent 0.72.)

Some diet book authors claim a food's GI and in some cases GL are the most important guidelines to use when planning a weight-loss diet. But consider the following: Pears (not shown in Table 17) are forbidden by some diets because of a relatively high GI = 40. However, a medium size pear weighing about four ounces has a GL = 4, quite low. Now consider a four ounce serving of peanuts with a much lower GI = 14, and an even lower GL = 2. For people on a reducing diet, based only on Glycemic Index or Load, a snack of peanuts appears to be a better choice than a pear. A medium-size pear, however, contains only 70 kcalories, while 110 grams of peanuts are loaded with about 650 kcalories! Pears and peanuts are both healthy foods, but the extra 580 kcalories in peanuts are certainly not going to help you lose weight.

The focus on a food's GI can lead to limiting healthful foods that may have a high GI by themselves, but when eaten in combination with other foods are not a problem. A nutritious baked potato may have a high GI, but when eaten as part of a complete meal is digested more slowly than its GI value would indicate. The main point is that if you use GI or GL values

Food	Glycemic Index	Serving Size	Net Ca	Glycemic
Strawberries	40	1 cup (150 g)	3	1
Peanuts	14	3.5 oz. (100 g)	9	1
Peach	42	large (120 g)	8	3
Carrot	92	large (80 g)	4	4
Lentils	28	1 cup (150 g)	15	4
Orange	48	medium (120	9	4
Watermelon	72	1 cup (120 g)	6	4
Apple	40	medium (138	15	6
Ice Cream	65	1 scoop (50 g)	10	7
Bread (whole	73	1 slice (30 g)	11	8
Grapes	46	4 oz. (120 g)	18	8
Bread (white)	70	1 slice (30 g)	13	9
Corn (sweet)	59	1 ear (80 g)	16	9
Banana	50	large (120 g)	24	12
Oatmeal	58	1 cup (234 g)	21	12
Sweet potato	50	medium (150	26	13
Spaghetti	45	6 oz. (180 g)	44	20
Potato (baked)	94	medium (150	22	21
Rice (brown)	50	4.5 oz. (130 g)	48	24
Raisins	64	1 box (60 g)	43	28
Rice (white)	72	4.5 oz. (130 g)	42	30
Candy bar	55	1 bar (113 g)	64	35
Glucose	100	(50 g)	50	50

Table 17: Glycemic Rank of Common Foods

as the sole factor when selecting your food, you could be eliminating very healthy foods, and eating too many calories and often too much fat as well. It is important, therefore, to appreciate that a food's GI and GL numbers only allow you to evaluate how a food's carbohydrate content affects your blood sugar. Because your body performs better when your blood sugar level remains relatively constant, you should be aware of a food's GL rank and consider it when planning your eating pattern. But there are other important factors that must be taken into account, such as getting the micronutrients you need from a variety of foods, including carbs, and staying within your caloric allowance.

In summary, **carbohydrates are neither all good nor all bad.** Remember good carbohydrates provide needed micronutrients. You should try to get the bulk of your calories from the good carbohydrates, i.e., from fruits, from vegetables and from whole grains such as whole-grain cereal, whole-wheat bread, whole-grain pasta, whole-old-fashioned oats, brown rice, bulgur, millet, and hulled barley.

Cholesterol and Triglyceride Levels

Atherosclerosis has been linked to both blood cholesterol and triglyceride levels. Both fatty substances are found in the plaque on the walls of clogged arteries. There are two types of cholesterol: high-density cholesterol (HDL), the "good" cholesterol, and low-density cholesterol (LDL), the "bad" cholesterol. You should have your cholesterol and triglyceride levels measured during a regular medical checkup and should know and understand the readings. At this writing, the desirable readings for otherwise healthy individuals are as follows:

- **Total cholesterol: less than 200 mg/dl.**
- **HDL cholesterol: greater than 40 mg/dl.**
- **LDL cholesterol: less than 130 mg/dl.**
- **Triglycerides: less than 150 mg/dl.**

For people who have coronary-artery disease, most cardiologists insist that the total cholesterol level be less than 160 mg/dl and the even more important LDL cholesterol be less than 100 mg/dl. Recently, cardiologists have been urging patients with coronary-artery disease to reduce their LDL even further to below 70 mg/dl.

Often, cholesterol and triglyceride levels can be reduced by adhering to the eating recommendations summarized at the end of the section that immediately follows, called "Fats in Foods." Where a low-fat diet alone does not work, people with high cholesterol and or high triglyceride levels, may be prescribed cholesterol-lowering medication by their physician. For more information on this important subject, visit the American Heart Association website: http://www.americanheart.org.

Fats in Foods

Fats are found in vegetable oil, seeds and nuts, meat and fish, and dairy products, as well as in foods like potato chips and French fries (that are cooked in oil), cookies, cake, and so on. There are certain fats you absolutely need to survive (the essential-fatty acids), and others you would do well to drastically limit (saturated fats) or avoid altogether (trans fats). Chemically, all fatty acids contain carbon chains with hydrogen atoms bonded to the carbon, and all fats have the highest calorie density – containing nine calories per gram (more on this later).

Until recently, the best wisdom was to eat a low-fat, low-cholesterol diet. This advice is now largely out of date. The latest research seems to show that the total amount of fat in the diet may not be linked with disease. **What really matters is the type of fat in your diet.**

Saturated Fats: When all carbon bonds of a fat molecule are filled with hydrogen, a fat is said to be saturated, i.e., saturated with hydrogen atoms. Most saturated fats are animal in origin and are solid at room temperature (good examples are butter and the fat in meats). Generally speaking, you should avoid or at least severely limit your intake of saturated fats because they can raise both your total and bad LDL blood cholesterol levels which increases your chances of getting heart disease.

When hydrogen atoms are missing along the carbon chain the fatty acids are called monounsaturated or polyunsaturated depending on their exact chemical structure.

Monounsaturated fats (also called omega-9 fatty acids) are liquid at room temperature and are known as oils. They are "good fats" and are derived from plant sources, such as vegetable oils, nuts, and seeds. In studies in which monounsaturated fats were eaten in place of carbohydrates, LDL blood cholesterol levels decreased and HDL cholesterol levels increased. Monounsaturated fats are found in high concentrations in canola, olive and peanut oils.

Polyunsaturated fats are also liquid oils at room temperature and in your refrigerator. They are "good fats" and are derived from plant sources, such as vegetable oils, nuts, and seeds. Again, research has demonstrated that when polyunsaturated fats were eaten in place of carbohydrates, LDL blood cholesterol levels decreased and HDL cholesterol levels increased. Polyunsaturated fats are found in high concentrations in sunflower, soybean and corn oils.

Essential-Fatty Acids are class of polyunsaturated fatty acids that our body cannot create. These fats must be obtained from the food you eat. Essential-fatty acids promote absorption of the fat-soluble vitamins A, D,

E, and K and are also thought to provide many disease-fighting benefits. Because essential-fatty acids are needed and our body cannot manufacture them, they must come from the food we eat. Essential-fatty acids fall into two groups: omega-3 and omega-6.

Omega-3 fatty acids are relatively hard to find. Foods high in omega-3 fatty acids are walnuts, tofu, flax seeds and oily fish (salmon, mackerel, sardines, trout and albacore tuna). Omega-3 fats are thought to be heart-protective. (The American Heart Association suggests that people with coronary-heart disease consult with their physician regarding the advisability of taking a fish-oil supplement.)

Omega-6 fatty acids, on the other hand, are more common, easier to find, and are in most oils including sunflower, soybean and corn oils.

Current thinking is that the consumption of omega-6 and omega-3 fatty acids should be in the ratio of 3:1, with about three omega-6 for one omega-3. Many Western diets, however, contain about 15:1, omega-6 to omega-3, which is not good for your health. Although you need omega-6, people generally eat too much of it and not enough omega-3 fat. The American Heart Association recommends that you eat fish (particularly fatty fish) two times a week, as a way to get a more appropriate quantity of omega-3 fatty acids in your diet.

Fat Type	Where found
Saturated	**Meat, poultry (especially the skin), dairy products, lard, coconut oil, palm oil, cocoa butter**
Trans Fats	**Fried foods, margarine, snack foods, commercially-baked cake and cookies, and fast foods**
Cholesterol	**Egg yokes, dairy products, organ meats, fatty and prime meats, poultry skin, shellfish (particularly shrimp)**
Polyunsaturated (Omega-3)	Mackerel, salmon, sardines, tuna, canola oil, walnuts, flaxseed, wheat germ
Polyunsaturated (Omega-6)	Corn oil, cottonseed oil, safflower oil, sunflower oil, soybean oil
Monounsaturated (Omega-9)	Canola oil, olive oil, safflower oil (hybrid), sunflower oil (hybrid)

Table 18: Fats in Foods

Trans fats are produced when a liquid oil is processed into a solid fat. The manufacturing process is called hydrogenation, or partial hydrogenation, and trans fats are an unnatural by-product. Partially-hydrogenated vegetable oils are considered especially unhealthy, because of the resulting trans-fatty acids and the added hydrogen saturation. Research indicates that trans fats are even worse than saturated fats because they not only raise bad LDL cholesterol but also lower good HDL cholesterol. Eliminating foods containing partially-hydrogenated oils from your diet is vital to good health.

In summary, it is becoming increasingly clear that saturated and trans fats, increase the risk for certain diseases while monounsaturated and polyunsaturated fats, lower the risk. The key is not to eliminate fat from your diet but to substitute good fats for bad fats, and at the same time try to reduce the total amount of fat consumed because all fats are very high in calories. The current scientific thinking regarding fat consumption is as follows:

1) Try to limit the total fat you eat to no more than 30 percent of your caloric intake.

2) Do not consume foods containing partially-hydrogenated vegetable oil because they are high in trans fats. This includes commercially prepared baked goods, snack foods, and processed foods, including fast foods. To be on the safe-side, assume these food products contain trans fats unless labeled otherwise.

3) Limit saturated fats, i.e., any fat of animal origin, to 10 percent of your caloric intake. Have meat less often, and when serving meat use lean cuts and trim the fat. Eat fish and poultry (white meat, without the skin) more frequently. Use fat-free or low-fat-milk dairy products in place of whole-milk dairy products. (Coconut and palm oil should also be avoided because they are saturated fats.)

4) When consuming fat, choose foods containing monounsaturated fats like olive oil and canola oil, and foods rich in polyunsaturated omega-6 and omega-3 fatty acids.

5) Try to balance your intake essential fatty acids by eating more omega-3 fatty acids, found in walnuts, tofu, certain seeds and oily fish such as salmon, sardines and tuna.

Vitamins and Minerals

The following is a listing of vitamins and minerals complete with a brief discussion of their function in your body, what foods supply the particular micronutrient, and the Recommended Dietary Allowance (RDA) - which is a reference number developed by the United States Food and Drug Administration to help consumers determine how much of a specific micronutrient a food contains. Summaries of the RDAs for vitamins and minerals are shown in Table 19 (on page 69) and Table 20 (on page 73). Notice that RDAs are frequently gender and age dependent.

Because of the rapid expansion of scientific knowledge regarding the role of micronutrients in human health, the U.S. Food and Drug Administration, in partnership with Health Canada, periodically assesses and updates the recommended Daily Values. The following contains the recommended RDAs as of April 2016 for the vitamins and minerals discussed.

Table 19: RDA for Selected Vitamins

Vitamin	Men		Women	
	51-70	70+	51-70	70+
A (mcg)	900	900	700	700
D (mcg)	10	15	10	15
E (mcg)	15	15	15	15
K (mcg)	120	120	90	90
C (mg)	90	90	75	75
B_1 (mg)	1.2	1.2	1.1	1.1
B_2 (mg)	1.3	1.3	1.1	1.1
B_3 (mg)	16	16	14	14
B_5 (mg)	5	5	5	5
B_6 (mg)	1.7	1.7	1.5	1.5
B_7 (mcg)	30	30	30	30
B_9 (mcg)	400	400	400	400
B_{12} (mcg)	2.4	2.4	2.4	2.4

Values for vitamins D, K, B_5 and B_7 are "Adequate Intake."

like spinach, collards and romaine lettuce; and orange-colored fruits such as mango, cantaloupe and apricots; and red peppers and tomatoes. One medium-size carrot supplies approximately 270 percent of your RDA.

Vitamin D is a fat-soluble vitamin. Briefly, vitamin D is important in assisting the absorption of calcium, in forming strong bones and teeth and preventing deficiency diseases such as rickets and osteomalacia. For most adults, an adequate intake of vitamin D is 200 to 600 IU (which is equivalent to 5 to 15 mcg per day). In addition, your body can make vitamin D after exposure to sunshine. Good food sources include salt-water fish such as herring, salmon, sardines and fish-liver oils, as well as fortified milk and cereals. A 250 mL glass of fortified milk supplies about 25 percent of your daily needs.

Vitamin E is a fat-soluble vitamin that is a powerful antioxidant and acts to protect cells against the effects of free radicals, which are potentially damaging by-products of energy metabolism. Research is underway to determine if vitamin E, through its ability to limit the production of free radicals, might help prevent or delay the development of cardiovascular disease and some cancers. For adults, the RDA for vitamin E is 22.5 IU (as d-alpha-tocopherol) which is equal to 15 mcg per day. Foods rich in vitamin E are vegetable oils, nuts, seeds, milk fat, egg yolks, liver, dark-green-leafy vegetables, and whole-grain foods. Approximately 12 almonds provide 100 percent of your RDA for vitamin E.

Vitamin K is another fat-soluble vitamin, and is known as the clotting vitamin because without it blood would not clot. Some studies also indicate that it helps maintain strong bones in the elderly. Adequate intake of vitamin K for men is 120 mcg per day and for women 90 mcg per day. Good sources are dark-green-leafy vegetables, soybean, cottonseed, canola, and olive oil. People who eat these foods as part of a balanced diet should easily get enough vitamin K.

Vitamin C is a water-soluble, antioxidant vitamin. It is important in forming collagen, a protein that gives structure to bones, cartilage, muscle, and blood vessels. Vitamin C also aids in the absorption of iron, and helps maintain capillaries, bones, and teeth. The RDA for vitamin C is 90 milligrams (mg) per day for men and 75 mg per day for women. Foods rich in vitamin C are citrus fruits and juices, kiwifruit, strawberries, cantaloupe, broccoli, peppers, tomatoes, cabbage potatoes, and dark-green-leafy vegetables. A 180 mL glass of orange juice supplies 100 percent of a man's RDA.

Vitamin B is actually a complex of different water-soluble vitamins that often exist in the same foods. They perform an important role in our metabolism, in maintaining muscle tone along our digestive tract and in the health of our nervous system, skin, hair, eyes, mouth, and liver. The B complex vitamins are: vitamin B_1 (thiamine), vitamin B_2 (riboflavin), vitamin B_3 (niacin), vitamin B_5 (pantothenic acid), vitamin B_6 (pyridoxine), vitamin B_7 (biotin), vitamin B_9 (folic acid), and vitamin B_{12}

(cyanocobalamin). Many cereals are fortified with all the B vitamins. Depending on the brand, one serving of a fortified cereal provides from 25 to 100 percent of the RDA for all the B vitamins (except vitamin B_7 biotin).

Vitamin B_1 (thiamine) plays a vital role in the proper operation of your nervous system. Your body also needs B_1 to convert carbohydrates into sugar and then energy. The RDA for men is 1.2 mg per day and 1.1 mg per day for women. Vitamin B_1 is found in meat, wheat germ, whole-grains cereals and breads, in enriched cereals and breads, in beans, nuts and seeds, and in dark-green-leafy vegetables.

Vitamin B_2 (riboflavin) also has a crucial role in certain metabolic reactions, particularly the conversion of carbohydrates into energy. Riboflavin is also an important antioxidant. The RDA is 1.3 mg per day for men and 1.1 mg per day for women. The best sources of riboflavin are brewer's yeast, almonds, organ meats, whole grains, wheat germ, wild rice, mushrooms, soybeans, milk, yogurt, eggs, broccoli, and spinach. In addition, flour and cereals are often fortified with riboflavin.

Vitamin B_3 (niacin) helps clear toxic and harmful chemicals from your body. It also assists in the production of various hormones. Niacin improves your circulation and reduces blood cholesterol levels. The RDA is 16 mg per day for men and 14 mg per day for women. Foods containing significant amounts of niacin are liver, meat, poultry, fish, whole-grains and nuts.

Vitamin B_5 (pantothenic acid) is necessary for a variety of life-sustaining tasks such as generating energy from food, synthesizing essential fats, and the function of your adrenal glands. Adequate intake of vitamin B_5 for adults is 5 mg per day. Good sources include organ meats, eggs, fish and shellfish, poultry, soybeans, beans, dairy foods, avocado, and mushrooms.

Vitamin B_6 (pyridoxine) is needed for protein and red-blood cell metabolism. Your body also requires vitamin B_6 to make hemoglobin. For men and women up to 50 years old, the RDA is 1.3 mg per day. After 50, the RDA increases to 1.7 mg per day for men and 1.5 mg for women. Vitamin B_6 is found in a wide variety of foods including fortified cereals, beans, meat, poultry, fish, and some fruits and vegetables.

Vitamin B_7 (biotin) functions as a coenzyme in the synthesis of fat, glycogen and amino acids. An adequate intake of biotin is 30 mcg per day. A varied diet should provide enough biotin for most people. Liver, yeast and egg yokes are particularly rich food sources. It is also found in smaller amounts in fruit, meat and cheese.

Vitamin B$_9$ (folate or folic acid) helps produce and maintain new cells which is particularly important during periods of rapid cell division and growth such as in infancy and during pregnancy. Folate is needed to make DNA and RNA, the building blocks of cells. It is also thought to prevent DNA changes that may lead to cancer. For most adults, the RDA of folate is 400 mcg per day. Of course, woman who are expecting or nursing need more folate. Cooked dry beans and peas, peanuts, oranges, dark-green-leafy vegetables and green peas are folate-rich foods.

Vitamin B$_{12}$ (cyanocobalamin) enables your body to manufacture healthy red-blood cells. It also assists in the transmission of electrical signals between nerve cells. The recommended dietary allowance is 2.4 mcg per day. Adults over age 50 and vegetarians who do not eat animal foods are often advised to get their vitamin B$_{12}$ from a supplement or from fortified foods. Vitamin B$_{12}$ is found in fortified cereals, meat, fish and poultry.

Calcium is a mineral with several important functions. Most of the calcium in your body is used to support the structure of your bones and teeth. A small amount of calcium is in your blood, muscle, and the fluid between your cells. Calcium is also needed for muscle contraction, blood vessel contraction and expansion, the secretion of hormones and enzymes, and sending messages through the nervous system. For most adults, adequate intake is 1000 mg per day. Foods rich in calcium are milk, yogurt, natural cheeses (such as cheddar, Swiss and mozzarella), canned fish with soft bones such as salmon and sardines, and dark-green-leafy vegetables. 250 mL of milk (whole or skim) contains 30 percent of your RDA.

Chromium is important in the metabolism of fats and carbohydrates and in controlling blood sugar levels. It is an activator of several enzymes needed to drive numerous chemical reactions necessary to life. For men and women up to 50 years old, an adequate intake of chromium is 35 and 25 mcg per day respectively. After 50, the recommended adequate intake drops to 30 mcg per day for men and 20 for women. Whole grains, ready-to-eat bran cereals, seafood, green beans, broccoli, prunes, nuts, peanut butter, and potatoes are rich in chromium. A 120 mL container of chopped broccoli provides about 35 percent of your chromium RDA.

Iodine is a basic component of the thyroid hormone that regulates your metabolic rate. Lack of iodine can cause a number of physical and mental abnormalities. RDA for adult men and women is 150 mcg per day. Iodized salt, sea food and plants grown in iodine-rich soil are good sources of iodine. 100 grams serving of cooked haddock contains about 125 mcg of iodine.

Iron is an important mineral that aids the transport of oxygen in your body and is also needed for the regulation of cell growth. An iron

72

deficiency limits oxygen delivery to cells, resulting in fatigue and decreased immunity. The RDA for iron is 8 mg per day for men and 18 mg per day for pre-menopausal women. Foods rich in iron are shrimp, clams, mussels, oysters, sardines, lean meats (especially beef), organ meats, turkey (dark meat), spinach, cooked dry beans, peas, lentils, and whole-grain breads and cereals. 100 grams of beef liver has approximately 50 percent of your iron RDA, and fortified cereals can provide from 50 to 100 percent of your RDA.

Mineral	Men		Women	
	51-	70+	51-	70+
Calcium (mg)	1200	1200	1200	1200
Chromium (mcg)	30	30	20	20
Copper (mcg)	900	900	900	900
Fluoride (mg)	4	4	3	3
Iodine (mcg)	150	150	150	150
Iron (mg)	8	8	8	8
Magnesium (mg)	420	420	320	320
Manganese (mg)	2.3	2.3	1.8	1.8
Molybdenum	45	45	45	45
Phosphorus (mg)	700	700	700	700
Potassium (mg)	4700	4700	4700	4700
Selenium (mcg)	55	55	55	55
Zinc (mg)	11	11	8	8

Table 20: RDA for Selected Minerals

Values for calcium, chromium, fluoride & manganese are "Adequate Intake."

Magnesium is needed for hundreds of biochemical reactions in your body. It helps maintain normal muscle and nerve function, keeps heart rhythm steady, supports a healthy immune system, and keeps bones strong. The RDA is 420 mg per day for men and 320 for women. Dark-green-leafy vegetables, fish, some beans and peas, nuts and seeds, and whole grains are good sources of magnesium. 120 mL serving of cooked spinach has 75 mg of magnesium.

Phosphorus in combination with calcium is necessary for the formation of bones and teeth. Phosphorus is also involved in the metabolism of fats, carbohydrates and proteins, and in the effective utilization of many of the B vitamins. The RDA for adults is 700 mg per day. Rich sources of phosphorus are dairy products, meat, and fish. Phosphorus is also present in most soft drinks. Generally, a diet that provides adequate amounts of calcium and protein also provides a sufficient amount of phosphorus.

Potassium is involved in proper nerve function, muscle control and blood pressure regulation. (People engaged in vigorous exercise may need more potassium to replace that lost during exercise.) Low potassium levels can cause muscle cramping and cardiovascular irregularities. Adequate intake for men and women is 4700 mg per day. Potassium-rich foods include baked white or sweet potatoes, cooked leafy greens, winter (orange) squash, bananas, oranges, dried fruits (such as apricots and prunes), and cooked dry beans and lentils. A medium-size baked potato contains about 600 mg of potassium.

Selenium is an essential trace element that assists enzymes involved in antioxidant protection and thyroid hormone metabolism. The RDA is 55 mcg per day for men and women. The most important sources in American diets are meats, fish and grains. 100 grams of cooked cod provide about 32 mcg of selenium.

Zinc is an essential mineral that stimulates the activity of approximately 100 enzymes that promote biochemical reactions in your body. Zinc supports a healthy immune system needed for wound healing, and helps maintain your sense of taste and smell. The RDA for zinc is 11 mg per day for men and 8 mg per day for women. Oysters contain more zinc per serving than any other food. Other good sources are red meat, poultry, beans, nuts, certain seafood, whole grains, dairy products and fortified breakfast cereals which can provide from 50 to 100 percent of your RDA.

Phytonutrients

Phytonutrients are not vitamins or minerals. Rather they are the beneficial compounds that give fruits and vegetables their many colors. "Phyto" comes from the Greek word for "plant," and that is where phytonutrients are found – in plant foods such as fruits, vegetables, whole grains, dried beans, nuts and seeds. Unlike traditional macronutrients and micronutrients (protein, fat, vitamins and minerals), phytonutrients are not necessary for life; i.e., they are not required for normal metabolism and

their absence will not result in a deficiency disease. Despite this, research is expanding as evidence grows that phytonutrients have many beneficial qualities such as assisting the function of the immune system, reducing inflammation, acting directly against viruses, and playing a crucial role in preventing or reducing the risk of a number of
chronic ailments, including heart disease, diabetes and cancer.

One of the most important roles of phytonutrients is as an antioxidant. Free radicals, which are by-products of energy metabolism, can damage cells and are thought to contribute to the development of cardiovascular disease and cancer. When antioxidant molecules encounter free radicals they neutralize them – limiting the damage. Our body needs more antioxidants as we grow older, because our body's ability to repair itself diminishes with age. Antioxidants are also thought to help prevent cell damage by environmental carcinogens.

Scientists understanding of phytonutrients is still in its infancy. Despite this, about one thousand phytonutrients have been identified to date and with ever expanding research new compounds are continually being discovered and organized into classes. The best known phytonutrient classes are carotenoids and polyphenols.

Carotenoids are contained in the yellow, orange, and red pigment in fruits and vegetables, as well as in dark-green-leafy vegetables (where the usual yellow color is masked by the vegetable's green pigment)

Some of the phytonutrients within the carotenoids class are alpha-carotene (contained in carrots); beta-carotene (in broccoli, sweet potato, pumpkin and carrots); beta-cryptoxanthin (in citrus fruits, peaches and apricots); lutein (in leafy greens such as kale, spinach and turnip greens); lycopene (in tomatoes, tomato paste, guava, pink grapefruit and watermelon); and zeaxanthin (in green vegetables and citrus fruit).

Polyphenol compounds are natural components of a wide variety of plants. Foods rich in polyphenols include apples, red wine, red grapes, grape juice, strawberries, raspberries, blueberries, cranberries, onions, tea, and certain nuts. Polyphenols are further subdivided into flavonoids and nonflavonoids.

Some phytonutrients in the flavonoids subgroup are anthocyanins (in fruits); catechins (found in tea and red wine); flavanones (in citrus fruit) flavones (in most fruits and vegetables); flavonols (in most fruits, vegetables, tea and red wine); and isoflavones (in soybeans). The nonflavonoids subgroup contains ellagic acid (found in strawberries, blueberries and raspberries).

Guidelines for Healthy Eating

No single food can supply all the nutrients you need in the amounts you need. The most important factors in nutrition are variety, variety, variety! **Variety is the key to a nutritious diet**. As a means of setting strategies for food selection, the U.S. Department of Health and Human Services and the Department of Agriculture issue Dietary Guidelines every five years. The latest Dietary Guidelines recommend the following:

• **Make Half your Plate Fruits and Vegetables:** Eat red, orange, and dark-green vegetables, such as tomatoes, sweet potatoes, and broccoli. Eat fruit, vegetables, or unsalted nuts as snacks.

• **Switch to Skim or 1% Milk:** Both have the same amount of calcium and other essential nutrients as whole milk, but less fat and calories. If lactose intolerant, try calcium-fortified soy products as an alternative to dairy foods.

• **Make at least Half your Grains Whole:** Choose 100% wholegrain cereals, breads, crackers, rice, and pasta. Check the ingredients list on food packages to find whole-grain foods.

• **Vary your Protein Food choices:** Twice a week, make seafood the protein on your plate. Eat beans, a natural source of fiber and protein. Keep meat and poultry portions small & lean.

• **Choose Foods and Drinks with little or No Added Sugars:** Drink water instead of sugary drinks. Select fruit for dessert. Eat sugary desserts less often. Choose 100% fruit juice instead of fruit-flavored drinks.

• **Look Out for Salt (sodium) in Foods you Buy:** Compare sodium in foods like soup, bread, and frozen meals and choose the foods with lower numbers. Add spices or herbs to season food without adding salt.

• **Eat Fewer Foods that are High in Solid Fats:** Make major sources of saturated fats – such as cakes, cookies, ice cream, pizza, cheese, sausages, and hot dogs – occasional choices, not everyday foods. Select lean cuts of meats or poultry and fat-free or low-fat milk, yogurt, and cheese. Switch from solid fats to oils when preparing food.

• **To Maintain a Healthy Weight:** Basically enjoy your food, but eat less. Stay within your personal calorie limit. (Note that caloric needs will be covered in a later chapter.) Think before you eat: Is it worth the calories? Avoid oversized portions. Use a smaller plate, bowl, and glass. Stop eating when you are satisfied, not full.

• **Know your personal Daily Calorie Limit:** Keep that calorie number in mind when deciding what to eat. (Again, caloric needs will be covered in a later chapter.) Use a food log to keep track of how much you eat.

- **When Eating out Check posted Calorie Amounts:** Choose lower calorie menu options. Select dishes that include vegetables, fruits, and/or whole grains. Order a smaller portion or share when eating out. Cook more often at home, where you are in control of what's in your food.
- **If you Drink Alcoholic beverages, do so Sensibly:** Limit should be 1 drink a day for women or to 2 drinks a day for men.

Basic Food Groups

In this section we describe the various food groups, indicate what constitutes a serving size, and focus on the best foods within each group. (The foods in **bold font** are generally the most nutrient-dense foods – the best of the best.)

Fruit Group: Includes fresh, frozen, canned and dried fruits and fruit juices. Usually, <u>one serving</u> consists of approximately 130 grams of fresh, frozen or canned fruit, or 75 grams of dried fruit, or 250 mL of 100 percent fruit juice. This group can be divided further into citrus fruits, berries and grapes, and other fruits.

Citrus fruits: There are many excellent citrus choices including **oranges, grapefruit, lemons, limes, kiwifruit and kumquats**. All are low calorie foods that contain a negligible amount of fat and cholesterol, are high in vitamin C, and most have significant amounts of vitamin A, potassium and dietary fiber.

Berries & grapes: Among the fruits in this grouping are **blackberries, bilberries, blueberries, raspberries, strawberries, cranberries, gooseberries, purple grapes, black currents, raisins, and cherries**. Every fresh berry and grape is low calorie, with no fat or cholesterol, and all have small amounts of multiple micronutrients and a fair amount of dietary fiber. (Strawberries are also rich in vitamin C.) Some researchers claim that the blue and black-colored berries are packed with more disease-fighting antioxidants than any other fruit or vegetable. Of course, dark-red and purple grape contain the phytonutrient flavonol, the same antioxidant believed to give red wine its heart-protecting benefits.

Other fruits: This large subgroup includes a number of healthy foods such as **apples, apricots, bananas, cantaloupe, figs, mangos, papayas, peaches, pears, pineapples, plums, prunes and watermelon**. Again, most are low calorie, contain no fat or cholesterol, and are loaded with vitamins, minerals and phytonutrients. In addition, apples, apricots, figs, peaches, pears, pineapples, plums, prunes are good sources of dietary fiber. Cantaloupe is also high in vitamin C and watermelon contains the phytonutrient lycopene.

Vegetable Group: Includes fresh, frozen, dried and canned vegetables and vegetable juices In general, <u>one serving</u> from the vegetable group consists of about 130 grams of raw or cooked vegetables, or 250 mL of vegetable juice. This group can be broken down further into dark-green-leafy vegetables, orange-colored vegetables, starchy vegetables and other vegetables.

Dark-green-leafy vegetables: Every food in this category (which includes **bok choy, collard greens, kale, mustard greens, romaine lettuce, spinach, Swiss chard and turnip greens**) is low calorie with no fat or cholesterol, and is packed with micronutrients, especially vitamins A and C, calcium, iron, potassium and folate, as well as dietary fiber.

Orange-colored vegetables: The best in this subgroup are **carrots, orange-bell peppers, pumpkin, sweet potatoes, yams and winter squash**. All have negligible fat and cholesterol and are high in vitamin A, potassium and dietary fiber.

Starchy vegetables: This grouping overlaps somewhat with the orange-colored vegetable subgroup and the grains group. Among the foods included are **white potatoes, sweet potatoes, yams, yellow corn, and brown rice**. These vegetables are generally high in complex carbohydrates, B vitamins, potassium and dietary fiber.

Other vegetables: This extensive category contains **asparagus, broccoli, Brussels sprouts, cabbage, cauliflower, celery, cucumber, fennel, green beans, parsley, and summer squash**. The preceding are low calorie foods that contain a negligible amount of fat and cholesterol, and most have significant amounts of vitamins A and C, potassium, calcium, iron, other micronutrients and dietary fiber. Also in this category are **eggplant, garlic, leeks, onions and mushrooms** which contain few calories, no cholesterol, and important amounts of potassium, calcium, iron and other micronutrients, as well as dietary fiber. **Red peppers and tomatoes** are low-calorie vegetables with no cholesterol that are loaded with vitamins A and C, iron and dietary fiber. Tomatoes also contain the phytonutrient lycopene. **Avocado and olives** contain some beneficial monounsaturated and polyunsaturated fat, but no cholesterol. Avocados are relatively high in potassium and vitamin A, while olives have significant amounts of iron and calcium.

Grains Group: Includes all foods made from wheat, rice, oats, cornmeal and barley, such as bread, pasta, oatmeal, breakfast cereals and grits. <u>One serving</u> from the grains group consists of approximately 30 grams of bread (one thin slice), or 30 grams of ready-to-eat cereal, or 75 grams of cooked rice, pasta or cooked cereal. <u>At least half of all grains you eat should be</u>

whole grains. Grains are the seeds of varied grasses grown for food. The outermost layer of the grain is an inedible husk, called chaff. The next layer is the bran, a protective coating rich in fiber. When this layer is removed, the product is described as pearled or polished. Inside the bran is the endosperm (the starchy part of a grain) and the germ, the part highest in nutrients (e.g., wheat germ). Whole grains have all these components intact. Refined grains have the husk, bran, and germ removed. Many foods are a mixture of whole and refined grains. Check the ingredient list for the words "whole grain" or "whole wheat" to determine if a food is made from a whole grain. In the United States, to be labeled "whole grain" a food must contain more than 51 percent whole grain by weight.

Whole grains include: **barley, buckwheat, bulgur, corn, millet, oats, brown rice, rye, wheat and wild rice**. Some whole-grain foods are: **whole-wheat bread, whole-grain ready-to-eat cereal, whole-wheat crackers, oatmeal, popcorn, whole-wheat pasta**, and whole barley (in beef-barley soup). All grains are low in fat and contain no cholesterol. Whole grains are good sources of complex carbohydrates and dietary fiber, as well as several B vitamins (thiamin, riboflavin, niacin, and folate), vitamin E, and minerals (iron, magnesium, and selenium).

Meats, Beans (and nuts) Group: Generally, One serving from this group consists of about 30 grams of lean meat, poultry, or fish, or one egg, or 20 grams of shelled seeds, or nuts (including peanut butter), or 30 grams of cooked dry beans. This group can be divided further into subgroups consisting of meat and foul, fish, eggs, beans, and nuts and seeds.

Meat and Foul: **Skinless white-meat chicken and turkey** are relatively low calorie, low fat, low cholesterol foods that are powerful sources of high-quality protein, vitamin B_6, riboflavin, niacin, phosphorus and potassium. Most meats, even **lean meats**, are higher in fat and calories than chicken and turkey, but meats do provide high-quality protein and some important nutrients such as iron and B-vitamins.

Fish: Most fish are good choices including **cod, halibut, herring, mackerel, salmon, sardines, scallops, shrimp, snapper, trout and tuna**. Nearly all fish contain high levels of essential-fatty acids. (Oily cold-water fish such as wild salmon, sardines, herring, mackerel and tuna are high in omega-3 essential-fatty acid. Trout also has comparatively high omega-3 content.) All fish are relatively low-calorie foods and are good sources of the fat-soluble vitamins A and D. (Fish-liver oils have high levels of fat soluble vitamins, and have been used as dietary supplements for many years.) Nutritionally, seafood is better known for its dietary minerals than for its vitamins. This is because some minerals in fish, such as iodine and selenium, are not available at the same levels in most other non-marine foods. Fish are also a good source of iron and potassium.

There is, however, a downside to eating fish. Some fish are contaminated with mercury, PCBs, dioxins and other environmental pollutants. Mercury is a toxic heavy metal that can accumulate in certain fish species. Large predatory fish such as shark, swordfish, king mackerel and tilefish have the highest concentration of mercury and other environmental contaminates. Canned white albacore tuna, a commonly eaten fish, contains higher levels of mercury than canned light tuna. The U.S. Food and Drug Administration advises adults to eat no more than 180 grams of high-mercury fish per week.

PCBs are potential human carcinogens that find their way into fresh waters and oceans where they are absorbed by fish. A recent study reported that PCB levels in farmed salmon, especially those in from Europe, were about seven times higher than in wild salmon.

For further information about the safety of fish you catch locally, visit your local health department. If no advice is available, eat no more than 180 grams per week of fish caught from local waters and do not consume any other fish that week. According to the University of Michigan Integrative Medicine Department, pregnant and nursing women, and young children, should avoid shark, swordfish, king mackerel and tilefish, and strictly limit the amount of other contaminated fish consumed.

Eggs: Current dietary guidelines and the latest research concerning egg consumption appear to be at odds. On the one hand, because a typical egg yoke contains saturated fat and 300 mg of cholesterol, the latest dietary guidelines recommend that egg yolks and whole eggs be used in moderation (up to one egg per day), but that egg whites and egg substitutes can be used freely since they contain no cholesterol and little or no fat.

On the other hand, others argue that if judged as a whole food and not simply as a source of cholesterol, positives such as the fact that eggs are low calorie, are loaded with high-quality protein, are a good source of vitamin E, etc, are apparent. Moreover, researchers at the Harvard Medical School studied egg consumption among 120,000 nurses and other health professionals with normal cholesterol levels and reported no link between eating eggs and heart disease or stroke.

Some medical researchers advise that, if one is at low risk (i.e., does not smoke, exercises regularly, eats a healthy diet and has no family history of heart disease or stroke) and chooses to begin eating eggs, they should have a blood test four to six weeks after they start eating eggs to determine the impact on their total and LDL cholesterol. Based on the test results, you and your doctor can decide – yes or no to eating more eggs.

Beans: Among the foods in this important subgroup are **black beans, cannelloni beans, dried peas, fava beans, garbanzo beans, red kidney beans, lentils, lima beans, navy beans, and pinto beans**. All beans are inexpensive, low-fat, plant-protein-rich foods that are good sources of B vitamins, potassium, iron, dietary fiber and isoflavones (important phytonutrients).

Nuts and Seeds: This category consists of **almonds, cashews, hazelnuts, peanuts, pecans, pistachio nuts, walnuts, flaxseed, pumpkin seeds, sesame seeds, sunflower seeds**, and others. Because nuts and seeds contain significant amounts of essential-fatty acids, they are comparatively high-calorie foods. Most nuts and seeds have a good amount of dietary fiber, vitamin E, potassium, iron and folate. Almonds, cashews, peanuts, and pine nuts contain a significant quantity of plant protein and essential-fatty acids. Walnuts, flaxseed and pumpkin seeds are important sources of plant-based omega-3 fatty acids.

Soy: The soybean is the most widely grown legume. Healthful soy foods such as **tofu, soy nuts, soymilk, soybean oil, and soy protein** are made from soybeans. All contain a significant amount of plant-based <u>complete protein</u> and omega-3 fatty acid as well as vitamin E, potassium, iron and folate. Soy nuts are also high in dietary fiber.

Soybeans, tofu, and other soy-based foods are an excellent alternative to red meat. But there are some suspected dangers from too much soy. So do not to overdo it. The Harvard University School of Public Health recommends two to four servings of soy foods per week as a good goal. Furthermore, they caution adults not to take supplements that contain concentrated soy protein or soy extracts, such as isoflavones.

Milk Group: Includes liquid milk and all products and foods made from milk such yogurt and cheese. (Foods that have little or no calcium such as cream, butter and cream cheese are not in this group.) <u>One serving</u> from the milk group consists of 250 mL of milk or yogurt, or 40 grams of natural cheese, or 60 grams of processed cheese.

Milk, yogurt and natural cheeses are high in calcium and protein. **Milk** is also often fortified with vitamin D. In addition to calcium and protein, **yogurt** is a particularly wholesome food providing live active bacteria cultures which promote gastrointestinal health. Most choices in this group should be fat free or low fat.

Oils Group: Includes vegetable oils and foods such as **nuts, olives, oily fish, avocados**, mayonnaise, soft margarine and some salad dressings.

You should limit the intake of saturated fats – that is any fat of animal origin.

The oils group overlaps somewhat with many of the others. Liquid oils, however, are unique to this group. **Corn oil, flaxseed oil, safflower oil, sesame oil, soybean oil and sunflower oil** are polyunsaturated; whereas, **canola oil, olive oil and peanut oil** are monounsaturated. All these oils are high in calories and essential-fatty acids. Essential-fatty acids promote absorption of the fat-soluble vitamins A, D, E, and K. Flaxseed, canola and soybean oil contain omega-3 fatty acids. (Note, when purchasing olive oil, choose an oil that is labeled "extra-virgin" or "virgin." Virgin olive oils are produced from the first pressing of the olives, are unrefined and as a result are more healthful.)

Vitamin/Mineral Supplements

Even though most adults can get all the vitamins and minerals they need by merely consuming a variety of nutritious foods (from the fruit group, the vegetable group, the grains group, the meat and beans group, the milk group, and the oils group), **many physicians recommend a daily multi-vitamin/mineral supplement as a kind of insurance policy.**

Be aware that some micronutrients, such as the fat-soluble vitamin A, can be harmful if taken in large quantities. To be safe your multi-vitamin/mineral supplement should contain no more than 100 percent of the recommended dietary allowance (RDA) for each vitamin or mineral. Generally, you don't need the high doses in multi-vitamin/mineral supplements labeled "therapeutic" or "extra-strength." There may be medical reasons for taking larger amounts of a vitamin or mineral than the RDA provides, but check with your doctor first. For example, a physician may advise a pregnant woman to take an iron supplement, and women who could become pregnant to take folic acid in addition to consuming folate-rich foods to reduce the risk of some serious birth defects. Adults over age 50 and vegetarians who do not eat animal foods may be advised to get their vitamin B_{12} from a supplement or from fortified foods. Women with little exposure to sunlight may need a vitamin D supplement, and individuals who seldom eat dairy products or other rich sources of calcium may need to take a calcium supplement.

Dietary supplement choices include not only vitamins and minerals, but also herbal products and many other widely available substances. Herbal products, however, usually provide only small amounts of vitamins and minerals and their health value is currently being studied.

Organic Food – Yes or No?

Buying organic fruits, vegetables, dairy, meat and poultry can cost as much as 50 to 100 percent more than conventional non-organic foods. Is organic worth the extra cost? Read on.

"Organic" refers to the methods farmers grow and process agricultural products, including fruits, vegetables, grains, dairy products and meat. Farmers who grow organic produce and meat don't use conventional methods to fertilize, control weeds or prevent livestock disease. As an example, rather than using chemical weed killers, organic farmers conduct sophisticated crop rotations and mulch to keep weeds at bay. Instead of synthetic pesticides organic farms use helpful insects and birds, mating disruption or traps to reduce pests and disease. In place of chemical fertilizers, organic farms employ natural fertilizers, such as manure or compost. Animals on organic farms eat organically grown feed, aren't confined 100 percent of the time and are raised without antibiotics or synthetic growth hormones.

Is Organic Worth the Cost?

Most organic food costs more than non-organic conventional food products. Higher prices are due to more expensive farming practices, tighter government regulations and lower crop yields. The question is are organic foods worth the extra cost? Critics argue that we're wasting our money because there's no proof that conventionally produced foods pose significant health risks.

Some studies have linked chemical weed killers, synthetic pesticides and synthetic growth hormones in non-organic food to everything from headaches to cancer to birth defects. This growing body of research shows that pesticides and other contaminants are more prevalent in the foods we eat, in our bodies, and in the environment than we thought – but quite a few experts maintain that the levels of these alien substances in non-organic foods are safe for most healthy adults. Some scientists are also worried about the antibiotics given to most farm animals. Many are the same antibiotics we humans rely on, and overuse of these drugs has already enabled bacteria to develop resistance to them, rendering them less effective in combating infection in humans.

Although the USDA certifies organic food, it doesn't claim that organic products are safer or more nutritious. Indeed, there is no conclusive evidence that shows that organic food is more nutritious than conventionally grown non-organic food.

In this writer's opinion, if you can afford it, buy local and organic, but you don't have to buy organic across the board because not all organic-labeled products offer added health value. For example, it's worth paying more for the "dirty dozen": peaches, strawberries, nectarines, apples, spinach, celery, pears, sweet bell peppers, cherries, potatoes, lettuce, and imported grapes. These fragile fruits and vegetables often require more pesticides to fight off bugs compared to hardier produce, such as asparagus and broccoli. But you can also pass on organic seafood and shampoo, which have labels that are often misleading.

You can also find organic food at most farmer's markets, and many of the farmers don't charge an organic premium. Another alternative is to buy a share in a community-supported organic farm. You'll get a weekly supply of produce from spring until fall. Costs are reasonable although most farms will require you to work a few hours a month distributing or picking produce. The cost savings can be substantial.

Is Vegetarianism for You?

A strict vegetarian diet is one that rejects all animal-based foods (including poultry, game, fish, shellfish or crustacean) and slaughter by-products. There are several variants of the diet. A generic term for both vegetarianism, veganism, and similar diets, is "plant-based" diets. The reasons for choosing a plant-based diet are varied and may be centered on morality, religion, culture, ethics, aesthetics, environment, society, economy, politics, taste, nutrition or health.

When deciding what type of vegetarian you might want to be, think about what foods you want to include or avoid. Understanding the following popular vegetarian types may help you decide.

1). Lacto-Ovo Vegetarians do not eat animal flesh of any kind (including beef, pork, poultry, fish and shellfish) but they do eat eggs and dairy products. Some ovo-lacto vegetarians eat meat by-products (e.g. fats, bone meal, gelatin) and use animal-derived products (leather etc.). This is the most practiced type of vegetarianism.

2). Lacto-Vegetarians do not eat animal flesh of any kind (including beef, pork, poultry, fish and shellfish) and do not eat meat or eggs – but do eat dairy products.

3) Ovo-Vegetarians do not eat animal flesh of any kind (including beef, pork, poultry, fish and shellfish) and do not eat meat or dairy products – but do eat eggs.

4). Semi-Vegetarians abstain from eating all meat and animal flesh with the exception of fish – although factory-farmed fish are usually avoided..

People are adopting this kind of diet, usually for health reasons or as a stepping stone to a fully vegetarian diet.

5). Vegans are strict vegetarians who do not eat meat of any kind and also do not eat eggs, dairy products, or processed foods containing these or other animal-derived ingredients. Many vegans also refrain from eating foods that are made using animal products even though the food may not contain animal products in the finished product, such as sugar and some wines.

Estimating Calorie Value of Foods

In order to plan a diet you must be able to estimate the calorie value of foods as well as portion sizes. The Nutrition Facts label on food packages, listing nutrient content, makes it possible to calculate the number of calories in a serving if you know that there are roughly:

	Calories per gram
Carbohydrates	4
Protein	4
Alcohol	7
Fat	9

Example Determine the calories in a cup 250 mL of whole milk. The label on a container of whole milk indicates that 250 mL has 11 grams of carbohydrate, 8 grams of protein and 9 grams of fat. The total calories in a cup of whole milk can be determined as follows:

11 gm carbs x 4 kcal per gm = 44 kcal
8 gm protein x 4 kcal per gm = 32 kcal
9 gm fat x 9 kcal per gram = 81 kcal
Total = 44+32+81 = **157 kcalories**

A sense of the **caloric value per 100 grams** of some basic foods are listed in Table 21 (on page 86). The extremes of the chart are represented by water the lowest, which has zero kcal and fat (lard) the highest at about 900 kcal per 100 grams. Sugar (a pure carbohydrate) is near the middle of the ranking at 400 kcal per 100 grams. (Note, protein is also approximately 400 kcal per 100 grams but there is no pure protein food to rank.) (Note, most of the calorie values in Table 21 are the average of many varieties in a particular category.)

Water	**0**	Pasta	125
Coffee or Tea	4	Fish	150
Vegetables	25	Eggs	163
Milk (fat free)	32	Poultry	187
Soft drink	42	Whiskey	249
Beer	44	Bread	270
Fruit	50	Meat	320
Milk (whole)	66	Cake	400
Potato	76	**Sugar**	**400**
Corn	87	Chocolate	530
Wine	88	Nuts	610
Rice	114	Vegetable oil	884
Beans	118	**Lard**	**900**

Table 21: kcalorie Rank of Basic Foods

Table 22 on page 88 is an expanded version of the Table 21 that includes the **kcalories per 100 grams** of some commonly encountered foods.

If you appreciate that **most foods are some combination of water, carbs, protein, fat and fiber**, this can lead to a better understanding of why a particular food has the caloric value and rank shown in Table 22. For example, watermelon is almost entirely water, with some fiber (zero calories) and carbohydrate, with no protein or fat, and consequently has a very low 26 kcalories per 100 g value. A grape is again mostly water with some fiber and carbohydrate and according to the chart has only 68 kcal per 100 g, but a raisin (a dried grape) is almost entirely carbohydrate and fiber with little water and thus has a value of 290 kcal per 100 g – closer to the 400 kcal per 100 g of a pure carbohydrate. When a food is not listed in the chart, common sense can often be used to estimate its caloric value; e.g., green beans are not listed, but judging from the ranking of similar foods a value of 25 or 30 kcal per 100 g seems reasonable.

Table 22 can also be thought of as a listing of the "caloric density" of foods. As an example, the table illustrates that one kilo of carrots contains about 360 kcal, or approximately the same number of calories as 100 grams of sirloin steak at 360 kcal. (Note that the numbers in the table are approximate kcalories per 100 grams of fluid or dry weight.)

Water	0	Peas	71	Liverwurst	278
Coffee/Tea	4	Yogurt (whole)	73	Hamburger	286
Vinegar	9	Potato (boiled)	76	Tuna (in oil)	288
Lettuce	15	Clams (raw)	79	Raisins	290
Celery	16	Banana	85	Bologna	304
Asparagus	23	Corn	87	Wheat Flakes	310
Tomato	24	Wine	88	Cake (average)	350
Spinach	25	Lobster	93	Sirloin Steak	360
Watermelon	26	Lentils	106	Cheese	370
Lemon	27	Scallops	112	Ham (baked)	370
Broccoli	28	Rice	114	Oatmeal	375
Mushrooms	30	Beans	118	Sugar	400
Cantaloupe	30	Pasta	125	Pretzels	390
Milk (fat free)	32	Tuna (in water)	127	Crackers	400
Carrots	36	Olives (black)	129	Doughnut	410
Strawberries	37	Blue Fish (baked)	159	Fudge	410
Green Pepper	37	Egg (boiled)	163	Chocolate	530
Peach	38	Turkey (light)	176	Potato Chips	568
Grapefruit	40	Ice Cream	193	Peanut Butter	585
Cola Drink	42	Sardines	196	Almonds	598
Beer	44	Turkey (dark)	203	Bacon	611
Yogurt (fat free)	44	Pancakes	225	Walnuts	630
Orange	50	Bread (wheat)	243	Butter	716
Apple	56	Whisky-86 proof	249	Mayonnaise	718
Milk (whole)	66	Apple Pie	256	Margarine	720
Cherries	68	Bread (white)	270	Vegetable Oil	884
Grapes	68	Jam/Jelly	272	Lard (fat)	900

Table 22: kcalorie Rank of Common Foods

Moreover, Table 22 in combination with a small weighing scale makes a very useful diet aide, allowing the calorie value of many food portions to be estimated quite accurately. It is a simple mater to weigh a piece of meat or a pancake, or a slice of apple pie, and multiply the weight in grams by the kcalorie value per 100 grams (from Table 22) to determine the total number of kcalories. Frequently, this approach will result in more precise calorie values than those obtained from the numbers shown in a common calorie table where the portion size is often ambiguously described.

You Need Fiber

Fiber is an important part of a healthy diet. **You need to consume fiber to assist your digestive system**. According to the Harvard University School of Public Health, adequate fiber intake reduces the risk of developing various conditions, including heart disease, diabetes, diverticular disease, and constipation.

Three fibers that are eaten on a regular basis are cellulose, hemicellulose and pectin. Hemicellulose is found in the hulls of different grains like wheat; e.g., wheat bran is hemicellulose. Cellulose is the structural component of plants, and gives vegetables their familiar shape. Pectin is found most often in fruits, is soluble in water but non-digestible, and is usually referred to as "water-soluble fiber." The best fiber sources are:

- **Whole-grain breads**, whole-grain cereals, whole-wheat pasta and brown rice contain a great deal of hemicellulose fiber.
- **Fruits** are pectin rich (the water-soluble fiber). The skin on fruits are loaded with phytonutrients and fiber. So do not peal an apple. Eat it with the skin on and get a fiber and nutrient boost.
- **Most berries** (such as bilberries, raspberries) have even more fiber than a comparable weight of most other fruit selections.
- **Vegetables** have lots of cellulose fiber. Again the skin is particularly high in fiber. When you eat a baked potato, eat it skin and all – everything – everything that is except the butter or sour cream.
- **Peas and beans** are high fiber foods that are also a complete protein when eaten with a whole grain food, or nuts, or seeds.
- **Nuts and seeds** add fiber to your diet.

When you eat fiber, in any of its forms, it simply passes straight through, untouched by but aiding your digestive system. Zero calories absorbed! Adults should get 20 to 35 grams of dietary fiber per day. The best sources are fresh fruits and vegetables, nuts and legumes, and whole-grains.

Drink Lots of Water

The average adult female body is about 52 percent water, while the average adult male body is approximately 63 percent water. If you are average, everyday you lose about 2500 mL of water when you breathe, perspire, and excrete waste. Because water is needed for almost every biochemical and physiologic process in your body, to maintain your body's water balance you must replace this lost water. (The water in your body is said to be balanced, when your water intake from all sources equals your loss of water.)

Typically, the food you eat every day contains about 750 mL of mostly concealed water. When you metabolize the food you eat, you create another 250 mL of water. That leaves about 1500 mL that must be replaced by the liquids you drink – more when you exercise. It appears, therefore, that the long-established wisdom advocating that you drink eight glasses of water per day (or any healthy beverage such as tea or fruit juice) is close to the mark.

Go Easy on Salt

Sodium and sodium chloride (salt) normally occur in small quantities in many natural foods. Salt and sodium-containing ingredients are also frequently found in high amounts in processed foods, such as canned soup and baked goods. People also add salt during food preparation and to the food they eat.

Although sodium plays an important role in your body, many studies have demonstrated that high sodium intake is also associated with high blood pressure. In your body, sodium retains water expanding blood volume which in turn raises blood pressure. Moreover, although some questions remain, evidence suggests that many adults who are predisposed to high blood pressure (for example having a parent who has high blood pressure) can reduce their chances of developing high blood pressure by consuming less sodium.

Most Americans consume too much sodium. The U.S. Department of Health and Human Services and the Department of Agriculture Dietary Guidelines recommend that healthy adults **limit sodium intake to 2400 mg per day.** (Note that one level teaspoon of salt contains about 2300 mg of sodium.) Individuals who have high blood pressure and are also salt sensitive are frequently advised to limit their sodium intake even further.

Restrict Sugar

Sugars are carbohydrates and come in many forms. Sugar is found naturally in fruits, some vegetables, milk, breads, cereals and grains, and is often added to foods during processing, preparation and when eating. Added sugar and naturally occurring sugars are chemically identical and your body cannot distinguish between them.

Cake, cookies, candy and many beverages contain large amounts of added sugar that supply a large number of "nutritionally-empty calories." Only very active people with high calorie needs can afford to consume any quantity of these sugar-laden foods. **Sugar should be used sparingly** by people with low calorie needs and in moderation by most other healthy adults. (Contrary to what many believe, the latest scientific evidence seems to indicate diets high in sugar do not cause diabetes. Rather, scientific evidence indicates that adult-onset diabetes occurs most often in those who are overweight.)

Limit Alcohol & Caffeine

Wine and beer contain a small amount of nutrients and micronutrients, but other alcoholic beverages, such as whiskey, vodka and gin consist of nothing but "nutritionally-empty calories." Because alcohol has effects that can also be harmful when consumed in excess, it is worth repeating: If you drink alcohol do so in moderation.

Some research has shown that moderate drinking is associated with a lower risk of coronary- heart disease, but high levels of alcohol intake also raise your risk for high blood pressure, stroke, heart disease, certain cancers, and of course accidents. Heavy drinking may cause cirrhosis of the liver, inflammation of the pancreas, brain damage, and in some cases malnutrition (because alcohol contains calories that are often substituted for those in more nutritious foods).

Caffeine should also be used in moderation. Caffeine is found in coffee, tea, some soft drinks and foods that contain cocoa. It is also in some drugs such as cold remedies and in medicine sold over the counter to relieve headaches.

About Sports Drinks

When you sweat, you lose both water and salt. An imbalance of any of the electrolytes in your body (such as sodium) can be harmful and even dangerous. You can make sure you're replacing the sodium you lose when you sweat during exercise by consuming a sports drink such as Gatorade.

And many endurance athletes do just that when participating in long events.

But this book is not for endurance athletes, it is a guide for those of us who typically workout moderately for an hour or less. In fact, the majority of exercise physiologists feel that sports drinks are unnecessary for most people, and that plain water, along with the salt in the food we eat, are all that is needed to replenish the water and sodium lost during **moderate exercise**.

Common Sense Nutrition

1) Know your daily caloric allowance whether you are trying to maintain your weight or are on a reducing diet. (More on this in the next chapter.)

2) Eat a variety of foods within your caloric allowance, and consult the **Basic Food Groups** to shape your eating patterns. Try to choose the proper quantity from each food group.

3) Try not to consume foods containing partially-hydrogenated vegetable
oil because they are high in trans fats. This includes commercially prepared baked goods, snack foods, and processed foods, including most fast foods.

4) Limit your intake of saturated fats. Eat meat less often and fish and poultry more often, and use fat-free milk and milk products.

5) When possible, select fresh and natural foods and whole-grain products, and avoid chemical preservatives and additives, artificial and imitation foods, refined and processed foods, and foods that are mostly "nutritionally-empty calories."

6) Eat nutritionally-dense foods rather than calorie-dense foods.

7) Take a daily multi-vitamin/mineral supplement.

8) Before you buy, **read and understand the labels on food packages.**

Eat Slowly

One final important point, try to **eat slowly**. This is especially vital if you are on a diet, trying to lose weight. If you are someone who eats fast, who finishes before everyone else at the table, you are not giving yourself a chance to feel full. While everyone else is still eating, you either sit there and pick, or you have seconds, taking in extra calories you could avoid if you would just slow down.

WEIGHT LOSS

In developed countries, approximately 70 percent of men and women over 65 years old are overweight. Because obesity and overweight are so common and public interest is so great, we are all continually assaulted by a blinding array of fad diets, miracle pills, health spas, exercise devices, reducing belts, and the like. Most people are left bewildered not knowing what to believe. The truth is that weight control, although a relatively complex issue, is governed by a set of logical, scientific principles, and the acceptance and understanding of these principles – augmented of course by desire and self-discipline – can lead you to sure and lasting weight control.

According to the well established, scientifically valid, conservation of energy principle, when the human body is in energy equilibrium, the energy value of the food consumed minus waste, equals the sum of the basal energy and the energy expended during physical activity. When the energy taken in equals the total energy expended, weight is neither gained nor lost. When there is an energy imbalance, however, weight is either gained or lost. In general, we can state:

- **Weight Gain** occurs when your food energy intake is greater than the total energy you expend. In this case your body stores the extra energy as fat.

- **Weight Loss** occurs when your food energy intake is less than the total energy you expend. In this case your body converts stored fat (and in some cases muscle) into energy.

The measure of energy, whether in the form of food, physical activity, or heat is the kilocalorie (hereafter simply called the Calorie). As mentioned previously, weight loss occurs when you eat fewer calories than the calories you use in daily living. This difference in calories is referred to as the calorie deficit. How much weight you lose depends on the magnitude of the calorie deficit. In technical terms, **the calorie deficit, or calorie difference, is the driving force for weight change**. (Techies will appreciate that the calorie deficit which is the driving force for weight change is somewhat analogous to a voltage difference which is the driving force for the flow of electricity, and to a temperature difference which is the driving force for the flow of heat.) Researchers have shown that whether you are trying to lose weight or just maintain your weight, it's calories that count. In theory it does not matter what foods the calories are from. Too much of any food can result in weight gain.

Simplified Weight Loss Math

As stated previously, weight loss occurs when your food energy intake is less than the total energy you expend. Again, this difference in calories is referred to as the calorie deficit. How much weight you lose depends on the magnitude of your calorie deficit.

People on any weight-loss diet invariably want to know how much weight they will lose – and how fast. Simple metabolic calculations make a rough estimate possible. Physiologists have long known that to lose one kilo requires a deficit of approximately 7700 kcalories. Therefore, if a person's total calorie deficit over time is known, their weight loss over time can be calculated.

As will be evident later, a 40 year-old male office worker, who weighs 75 kilos, expends about 2552 kcal in day-to-day living. (In other words, if this man eats about 2552 kcal per day he will neither gain nor lose weight.) If he goes on a 1500 kcal reducing diet, his daily deficit would be 2552 – 1500 = 1052 kcal. In one week his deficit would be 1052 kcal per day x 7 days = 7364 kcal, and he should lose 7364 / 7700, or slightly less than one kilo.

This computation technique, however, is somewhat crude. Primarily because it does not account for a very important scientific fact: **As you lose weight you actually need fewer calories to maintain your lower weight.** As a result, if your calorie intake remains constant over some period of time, your calorie deficit will decrease during your diet and the rate at which you lose weight also will decrease with time.

This computation technique, however, is somewhat crude. Primarily because the preceding calculation does not account for a very important scientific fact: **As we lose weight we actually need fewer calories to maintain our lower weight.** As a result, if a dieter's calorie intake remains constant over some period of time, their calorie deficit will decrease during their diet and the rate at which they lose weight will also decrease with time.

Weight Loss Prediction Tables

Fortunately, a more precise determination of the rate of weight loss is possible. Scientists have demonstrated that **weight loss is a function of age, sex, height, weight, physical activity, caloric intake and the duration of the diet (or time on the diet).** This writer related all these variables in a complex, scientifically based, energy-weight-control equation, published in the *American Journal of Clinical Nutrition,*, and subsequently published a set of 60 Weight Loss Prediction tables in hardcover book *The Computer Diet*. In this edition of *Senior Fitness* you will find an abridged set of 12 Weight Loss Prediction tables (Tables 24 through 35).

Selecting the Correct Table

Your first task is to choose the correct Weight Loss Prediction Table. The twelve Weight Loss Prediction Tables are organized by gender, age and activity level. The three activity levels most applicable to seniors are covered in this text:

1) **Sedentary**: Inactive most of the day with very little standing or walking.
2) **Relatively Inactive**: Seated most of the day with about four hours of standing and incidental walking.
3) **Moderately Active**: To qualify for this category, you have to engage in some form of regular exercise everyday (e.g., taking a brisk three-mile walk).

Use Table 23 to find the Weight Loss Prediction Table that is applicable to you. Note: in the tables that follow, "Relatively Inactive" and "Moderately Active" often have been shortened to "Inactive" and "Active."

Gender	Age	Activity Level	Table
Men	50 - 65	Sedentary	24 - page 97
	50 - 65	Inactive	25 - page 98
	50 - 65	Active	26 - page 99
	66 - 80	Sedentary	27 - page 100
	66 - 80	Inactive	28 - page 101
	66 - 80	Active	29 - page 102
Women	50 - 65	Sedentary	30 - page 103
	50 - 65	Inactive	31 - page 104
	50 - 65	Active	32 - page 105
	66 - 80	Sedentary	33 - page 106
	66 - 80	Inactive	34 - page 107
	66 - 80	Active	35 - page 108

Table 23: Weight Loss Prediction Tables

Weight Loss Prediction Example

Consider a 63-year-old woman who weighs 70 kg, is retired does some light house work but spends most of her free time watching TV. How long will it take her to lose 10 kilos?

First she should choose **Table 31** on page 104, labeled "Weight Loss Prediction for Relatively Inactive Women, Ages 50 - 65 years." Then she would scan the far left of the table and locate her present weight of 70 kg; from this number she would run a finger horizontally (to the right) until it intersects the vertical column headed by the 10-kg weight loss she desires. The three numbers at the intersection are the time in days to lose 10 kilos, depending on the diet calories consumed. Specifically, to lose 10 kilos our fictional female's diet calorie options are:
- 900 kcal per day for 68 days.
- 1200 kcal per day for 89 days.
- 1500 kcal per day for 130 days.

Which alternative should she choose? Health professionals recommend a gradual weight loss of about one kilo per week. In this case, that would mean her diet should last about 10 weeks or about 70 days, pointing to the 900-kcalorie diet option.

But it is difficult to get all the nutrients you need on 900 kcal and a 900 kcal diet is also difficult stay on because most people feel hungry on 900 kcal. So she chooses the longer duration 1200 kcal diet. Better still would be for this woman to increase her activity level by taking a brisk 5 km walk everyday and qualify for the moderately active category (Table 32) which would result in the following shorter-duration diet options:
- 900 kcal per day for 57days.
- 1200 kcal per day for 72 days.
- 1500 kcal per day for 96 days.

Hence, by increasing her activity level, she could decrease the time to lose the 10 kilos by 15 to 25 percent – depending on the diet-calorie level she chooses. Please note that the calorie allowance during a weight loss diet need not be the same for every day of the week. It's the average intake over an entire week that counts. For instance, if the woman in the previous example selects a 1500 kcal diet (which totals $1500 \times 7 = 10,500$ kcal for one week), and her eating pattern is such that she knows she will invariably eat more on weekends, she could plan for 1200 kcal on weekdays and 2250 on weekends. In effect, she would then be dieting on weekdays and eating "almost normally" on weekends. This eating pattern would amount to $(1200 \times 5) + (2250 \times 2) = 10500$ kcal per week, which is the same loss outcome as if she consumed 1500 kcal each and every day of the week.

Weight Loss Prediction for Men
(Sedentary - 51 to 65)

Present Weight	Diet kcal	Weight Loss (kg)							
		5	10	15	20	25	30	35	40
60 kg	1200	51				Numbers in table indicate time in days to lose weight.			
	1500	79							
	1800	177							
70 kg	1200	41	86						
	1500	58	124						
	1800	97	222						
80 kg	1200	35	72	113	159	209			
	1500	46	97	115	221	300			
	1800	68	147	244					
90 kg	1200	30	63	97	135	176	221	272	
	1500	38	80	126	177	235	301		
	1800	53	112	180	259				
100 kg	1200	27	55	86	118	153	190	231	277
	1500	33	69	107	149	195	246	304	
	1800	43	91	143	203	270	350		
110 kg	1200	24	50	77	105	136	167	203	240
	1500	29	61	94	129	168	209	255	306
	1800	37	77	120	167	220	279	347	
120 kg	1500	22	45	70	95	122	151	181	213
	1800	26	54	83	114	148	183	222	263
	2100	32	67	103	143	187	234	287	346
130 kg	1500	20	42	64	87	111	137	164	192
	1800	24	49	75	103	132	163	197	232
	2100	29	59	91	126	163	202	246	293

Table 24 Weight Loss, Men, 51 – 65

Weight Loss Prediction for Men
(Relatively Inactive - 51 to 65)

Present Weight	Diet kcal	Weight Loss (kg)							
		5	10	15	20	25	30	35	40
60 kg	1200	46							
	1500	68							
	1800	129							
70 kg	1200	37	78	124					
	1500	50	108	176					
	1800	78	175	304					
80 kg	1200	32	66	103	144	190			
	1500	41	86	136	194	261			
	1800	57	123	201	298				
90 kg	1200	28	57	89	123	160	201		
	1500	34	71	112	157	207	269		
	1800	45	95	152	218	296			
100 kg	1200	25	51	78	108	139	173	211	
	1500	30	61	96	133	173	218	269	
	1800	37	78	123	174	231	296		
110 kg	1200	22	45	70	96	124	153	185	219
	1500	26	54	84	116	150	187	228	273
	1800	32	67	104	145	190	240	297	
120 kg	1500	20	41	64	87	111	137	165	195
	1800	24	48	75	103	132	164	198	235
	2100	28	58	91	125	163	204	249	299
130 kg	1500	19	38	58	81	102	125	150	177
	1800	22	44	68	92	119	147	176	208
	2100	25	52	80	110	143	177	215	256

Numbers in table indicate time in days to lose weight.

Table 25 Weight Loss Men, 51 – 65

Weight Loss Prediction for Men
(Moderately Active - 51 to 65)

Present Weight	Diet kcal	Weight Loss (kg)							
		5	10	15	20	25	30	35	40
60 kg	1200	38				Numbers in table indicate time in days to lose weight.			
	1500	51							
	1800	80							
70 kg	1200	31	65	103					
	1500	39	84	135					
	1800	55	119	200					
80 kg	1200	26	55	86	120	157			
	1500	32	68	107	152	203			
	1800	42	89	144	209	289			
90 kg	1200	23	48	74	102	133	167	205	
	1500	27	57	90	125	165	209	260	
	1800	34	72	112	161	215	280		
100 kg	1200	21	42	65	90	116	145	176	210
	1500	24	50	77	107	139	175	214	259
	1800	29	60	94	132	174	221	275	340
110 kg	1200	19	38	59	80	103	128	154	185
	1500	21	44	68	94	121	151	183	219
	1800	25	52	81	112	146	184	225	229
120 kg	1500	17	35	53	73	93	115	138	163
	1800	29	39	61	83	107	133	161	190
	2100	22	46	71	98	127	127	192	229
130 kg	1500	16	32	49	67	85	105	125	147
	1800	18	36	55	75	97	119	143	169
	2100	20	41	63	87	112	139	168	199

Table 26 Weight Loss Men, 51 – 65

Weight Loss Prediction for Men
(Sedentary - 66 to 80)

Present Weight	Diet kcal	Weight Loss (kg)							
		5	10	15	20	25	30	35	40
60 kg	1200	57							
	1500	95			Numbers in table indicate time in days to lose weight.				
	1800	290							
70 kg	1200	45	96	153					
	1500	67	144	239					
	1800	125	298						
80 kg	1200	38	79	125	175	232			
	1500	52	110	176	254	349			
	1800	81	180	305					
90 kg	1200	33	68	106	147	193	243	300	
	1500	43	89	141	199	266	344		
	1800	61	130	212	310				
100 kg	1200	29	60	93	128	166	207	252	303
	1500	36	76	118	165	217	275	275	
	1800	49	103	164	234	315			
110 kg	1200	26	54	83	113	146	181	219	261
	1500	32	66	102	142	184	231	283	341
	1800	41	86	135	189	250	319		
120 kg	1500	24	49	75	102	131	162	195	230
	1800	28	59	90	125	161	200	243	290
	2100	36	74	115	160	65 209	263	324	
130 kg	1500	22	45	68	93	119	147	176	206
	1800	26	53	81	111	143	177	214	253
	2100	31	65	100	139	180	224	273	328

Table 27 Weight Loss Men, 66 – 80

Weight Loss Prediction for Men
(Relatively Inactive - 66 to 80)

Present Weight	Diet kcal	Weight Loss (kg)							
		5	10	15	20	25	30	35	40
60 kg	1200	51				Numbers in table indicate time in days to lose weight.			
	1500	79							
	1800	179							
70 kg	1200	41	86	137					
	1500	57	123	202					
	1800	95	219						
80 kg	1200	34	71	112	157	208			
	1500	45	96	153	219	298			
	1800	66	144	240					
90 kg	1200	30	62	96	133	175	219	270	
	1500	38	78	124	174	231	297		
	1800	51	108	175	252	348			
100 kg	1200	26	54	84	116	150	187	228	273
	1500	32	67	104	145	191	241	298	
	1800	43	88	138	196	262	340		
110 kg	1200	24	49	75	103	132	164	199	236
	1500	28	59	91	125	163	204	249	299
	1800	35	74	115	161	212	270	336	
120 kg	1500	22	44	68	93	119	147	177	208
	1800	25	52	81	111	143	178	215	256
	2100	31	64	99	138	179	225	276	333
130 kg	1500	20	40	62	85	108	133	159	187
	1800	23	47	72	99	126	158	190	225
	2100	27	56	87	120	156	194	236	281

Table 28 Weight Loss Men, 66 – 80

Weight Loss Prediction for Men
(Moderately Active - 66 to 80)

Present Weight	Diet kcal	Weight Loss (kg)							
		5	10	15	20	25	30	35	40
60 kg	1200	41				Numbers in table indicate time in days to lose weight.			
	1500	58							
	1800	97							
70 kg	1200	33	70	111					
	1500	43	93	151					
	1800	63	138	235					
80 kg	1200	28	59	92	129	170			
	1500	35	74	117	167	224			
	1800	47	100	162	238	335			
90 kg	1200	25	51	79	109	143	178	220	
	1500	30	62	97	136	179	228	286	
	1800	37	79	125	179	241	317		
100 kg	1200	22	45	69	95	124	154	187	224
	1500	26	53	83	115	150	189	232	282
	1800	31	65	103	144	191	244	307	
110 kg	1200	20	40	62	85	109	136	164	194
	1500	23	47	72	100	130	162	197	236
	1800	27	56	87	121	159	200	247	300
120 kg	1500	18	37	56	77	98	121	146	172
	1800	20	42	65	89	114	142	171	204
	2100	24	49	76	105	136	170	208	249
130 kg	1500	16	34	51	70	91	110	132	155
	1800	19	38	58	80	103	127	152	181
	2100	21	44	68	93	120	149	180	214

Table 29 Weight Loss Men, 66 – 80

Weight Loss Prediction for Women
(Sedentary - 51 to 65)

Present Weight	Diet (kcal)	Weight Loss (kg)							
		2	4	6	8	10	15	20	25
50 kg	900	20	41			Numbers in table indicate time in days to lose weight.			
	1200	31	64						
	1500	68	149						
55 kg	900	18	37	56					
	1200	26	54	84					
	1500	49	103	166					
60 kg	900	16	33	51	69	88			
	1200	23	47	72	99	128			
	1500	38	80	126	177	236			
65 kg	900	15	30	46	63	80	127		
	1200	20	41	64	87	112	181		
	1500	31	65	102	141	185			
70 kg	900	14	28	43	58	74	116	162	
	1200	18	37	57	78	99	1`59	228	
	1500	27	55	86	118	153	255		
80 kg	900	12	24	37	50	64	99	137	179
	1200	15	31	47	64	82	129	181	241
	1500	21	43	66	90	115	186	269	
90 kg	1200	11	22	33	44	56	87	120	155
	1500	13	27	41	55	70	109	152	199
	1800	17	35	54	73	93	147	208	279
100 kg	1200	10	20	30	40	51	77	107	138
	1500	12	24	36	49	62	95	132	171
	1800	15	30	46	62	78	123	172	226

Table 30 Weight Loss Women, 51 – 65

Weight Loss Prediction for Women
(Relatively Inactive - 51 to 65)

Present Weight	Diet (kcal)	Weight Loss (kg)							
		2	4	6	8	10	15	20	25
50 kg	900	18	38			Numbers in table indicate time in days to lose weight.			
	1200	27	56						
	1500	52	112						
55 kg	900	17	34	52					
	1200	23	48	74					
	1500	39	83	131					
60 kg	900	15	31	47	64	81			
	1200	20	42	64	88	114			
	1500	32	66	103	144	190			
65 kg	900	14	28	43	58	74	116		
	1200	18	37	57	78	100	160		
	1500	27	55	85	118	154	260		
70 kg	900	13	26	39	53	68	106	149	
	1200	16	33	51	70	89	142	203	
	1500	23	47	73	100	130	214		
80 kg	900	11	22	34	46	59	91	126	165
	1200	14	28	43	58	74	116	163	216
	1500	18	37	57	78	100	159	229	
90 kg	1200	10	20	30	41	52	80	110	143
	1500	12	24	37	50	63	99	137	179
	1800	15	31	47	64	81	128	181	241
100 kg	1200	9	18	27	37	47	72	98	127
	1500	11	21	33	44	56	86	119	154
	1800	13	26	40	54	69	108	150	197

Table 31 Weight Loss Women, 51 – 65

Weight Loss Prediction for Women
(Moderately Active - 51 to 65)

Present Weight	Diet (kcal)	Weight Loss (kg)							
		2	4	6	8	10	15	20	25
50 kg	900	16	32						
	1200	21`	44			Numbers in table			
	1500	34	72			indicate time in days			
55 kg	900	14	29	44		to lose weight.			
	1200	18	38	59					
	1500	27	57	90					
60 kg	900	13	26	40	54	69	13		
	1200	16	33	51	70	91	16		
	1500	23	47	74	102	185	23		
65 kg	900	12	24	36	49	63	99		
	1200	15	30	46	63	80	128		
	1500	20	41	63	86	112	185		
70 kg	900	11	22	33	45	57	90	126	
	1200	13	27	41	56	72	114	163	
	1500	17	36	55	75	96	157	260	
80 kg	900	9	19	29	39	50	77	107	140
	1200	11	23	35	47	60	94	132	174
	1500	14	29	44	60	76	121	173	233
90 kg	1200	8	17	26	35	44	68	94	121
	1500	10	20	30	41	52	81	112	146
	1800	12	24	37	50	63	100	140	185
100 kg	1200	8	15	23	31	39	61	83	107
	1500	9	18	27	36	46	71	98	126
	1800	10	21	32	43	54	85	118	154

Table 32 Weight Loss Women, 51 – 65

Weight Loss Prediction for Women
(Sedentary - 66 to 80)

Present Weight	Diet (kcal)	Weight Loss (kg)							
		2	4	6	8	10	15	20	25
50 kg	900	22	45						
	1200	36	74			Numbers in table			
	1500	95	217			indicate time in days			
55 kg	900	19	40	61		to lose weight.			
	1200	30	61	96					
	1500	62	133	219					
60 kg	900	18	36	55	75	96			
	1200	25	52	81	112	145			
	1500	46	97	155	221				
65 kg	900	16	33	50	68	87	137		
	1200	22	46	71	97	125	203		
	1500	37	77	121	169	225			
70 kg	900	15	30	46	62	79	125	175	
	1200	20	41	63	86	110	176	254	
	1500	31	64	99	138	179			
80 kg	900	13	26	40	54	68	106	147	194
	1200	17	34	52	70	89	141	199	266
	1500	23	48	74	101	130	212		
90 kg	1200	11	23	35	47	60	93	128	166
	1500	14	29	44	60	76	118	165	217
	1800	19	39	59	81	103	164	234	
100 kg	1200	10	21	31	42	54	83	113	146
	1500	13	25	39	52	66	102	142	184
	1800	16	33	50	68	86	135	189	250

Table 33 Weight Loss Women, 66 – 80

Weight Loss Prediction for Women
(Relatively Inactive - 66 to 80)

Present Weight	Diet (kcal)	Weight Loss (kg)							
		2	4	6	8	10	15	20	25
50 kg	900	20	41						
	1200	31	64			Numbers in table			
	1500	67	147			indicate time in days			
55 kg	900	18	36	56		to lose weight.			
	1200	26	53	83					
	1500	47	101	162					
60 kg	900	16	33	50	68				
	1200	22	46	71	98				
	1500	37	77	122	172				
65 kg	900	15	31	46	62	79	125		
	1200	20	41	62	85	110	178		
	1500	30	63	98	137	179			
70 kg	900	14	28	42	57	72	114	160	
	1200	18	36	56	76	97	155	223	
	1500	26	53	83	114	148	247		
80 kg	900	12	24	36	49	62	97	135	176
	1200	15	30	46	63	80	125	177	235
	1500	20	41	63	86	111	178	258	
90 kg	1200	10	21	32	43	55	85	117	152
	1500	13	26	39	53	68	106	147	193
	1800	16	34	51	70	89	141	200	267
100 kg	1200	9	19	29	39	50	76	104	134
	1500	11	23	35	47	59	92	127	165
	1800	14	29	43	59	75	117	164	216

Table 34 Weight Loss Women, 66 – 80

Weight Loss Prediction for Women
(Moderately Active - 66 to 80)

Present Weight	Diet (kcal)	Weight Loss (kg)							
		2	4	6	8	10	15	20	25
50 kg	900	17	34						
	1200	23	49			Numbers in table indicate time in days to lose weight.			
	1500	40	85						
55 kg	900	15	30	47					
	1200	20	41	64					
	1500	31	65	103					
60 kg	900	13	27	42	57	73			
	1200	18	36	56	76	98			
	1500	26	53	83	115	151			
65 kg	900	12	25	38	52	66	105		
	1200	16	32	49	67	86	139		
	1500	22	45	69	96	124	208		
70 kg	900	11	23	35	48	61	95	134	
	1200	14	29	44	60	77	123	176	
	1500	19	39	60	82	106	174	257	
80 kg	900	10	20	30	41	52	81	113	148
	1200	12	24	37	50	64	101	141	187
	1500	15	31	47	65	83	132	189	256
90 kg	1200	9	18	27	36	46	71	98	127
	1500	10	21	32	43	55	86	119	155
	1800	13	26	39	53	68	107	151	200
100 kg	1200	8	16	24	33	41	64	87	112
	1500	9	19	28	38	48	75	103	134
	1800	11	22	34	46	58	90	126	165

Table 35 Weight Loss Women, 66 – 80

Weight Loss Rate Will Decrease

It is well known that if your caloric intake on a weight-loss diet is constant, your rate of weight loss will decrease with time. In other words, as you lose weight it will get more difficult, or rather it will take a longer time to lose additional weight!

This declining weight loss rate is illustrated in Table 36 which shows weight loss versus the time on a 1500-kcalorie diet for a relatively inactive, 80 kg, 59-year-old female whose weight-loss goal is 55 kg. At the start of her diet, when she weighed 80 kilos, it took her **36 days to lose the first five kilos.**. The relevant Weight Loss Prediction (Table 31) for this person has been reconfigured for this example and shown as Table 36. Referring to Table 36, notice that the number of days between 5-kilo weight loss increments increased as she lost weight. In fact, toward the end of her diet, it took **53 days for her to lose the last five kilos** and reach her goal of 55 kg! Why does this happen?

To understand this phenomenon we have to temporarily move ahead to Weight Maintenance Table 42. (The Weight Maintenance tables list how many calories you can eat to neither gain nor lose weight.) From **Table 42** on page 131 we find that before she began her diet, she must have been consuming about 2436 kcalories per day to maintain her weight at 80 kg. At the start of her 1500-kcalorie diet, therefore, her deficit was 2436 – 1500 = 936 kcal per day, and she would have started losing weight at a rate of (936 x 7 / 7700), or 0.85 kilos per week.

At the end of her diet, the same table shows that at 55 kg she would have to eat no more than 1940 kcalories per day to neither gain nor lose weight. Her deficit would have been only 1940 – 1500 = 440 kcalories per day, and her weight lose rate would have dropped to (440 x 7 / 7700), or approximately 0.40 kilos per week.

Weight Loss	Time (days)	Data from Table 29
80 to 75 kg	36	
75 to 70 kg	38	(74 – 36 = 38)
70 to 65 kg	42	(116 – 74 = 42)
65 to 60 kg	47	(163 – 116 = 47)
60 to 55 kg	53	(216 – 163 = 53)

Table 36 Time to Lose the Next 5 kg

Weight Change Due to Water

When there is a calorie deficit the resulting weight loss is variable in its composition. Fat, water and protein (muscle, bone mass, etc) are lost at different rates at different times in the diet. Because water is often a significant component of weight loss, it is essential to understand how the amount of water in your body varies.

First, **realize that your body weight fluctuates two to three pounds daily - whether on a diet or not**. Your weight is lowest in the morning before breakfast and highest in the evening before retiring. In addition, the quantity of water in your body also varies from day to day. Over a reasonable period, however, the amount of fluid leaving your body will equal the amount entering your body by way of food and drink. The water balance of your body is then said to be in equilibrium.

At the start of any diet, there is usually a considerable loss of body water, and since 50 mL of water weighs about ½ kg, this initial water loss will appear to be a weight loss. But this weight loss is not "real" because only a small quantity of body tissue has been lost. (Many theories have been proposed to explain this phenomenon but none have been scientifically confirmed.) Changes in body hydration, therefore, cause a higher weight loss during the first week or so of a diet than is shown in the Weight Loss Prediction tables. By the following week, however, the body's water balance will again readjust and the total weight loss should more closely follow the values in the weight loss tables.

Another cause of weight fluctuation is water retention in women just prior to their menstrual period. (Not a concern for most senior women.) This water retention is not uncommon, but for the female dieter this may appear to be a time when weight is not lost. Again, the body's water balance will return to equilibrium the next week, when weight loss should once more closely follow the numbers in the Weight Loss Prediction table. The Weight Loss Prediction tables show "real" weight loss.)

The Dreaded Weight Loss Plateau

Many dieters complain that after losing some amount of weight, they get stuck; they reach a so-called "plateau," and stop losing weight – at least for some time period. If this happens to you, you will probably get discouraged and frustrated and wonder what you should do to break through and start losing weight again. Before we address solutions, let's examine the possible causes of a weight loss plateau.

First, you could actually still be losing weight but at such a such low a rate that your weight loss is masked by the natural daily fluctuations in your weight, and your perception is that you have reached a plateau. The low weight loss rate is no doubt due to the much lower calorie deficit associated with your new lower weight – as described in the previous section "Your Weight Loss Rate Will Decrease." Recall, as you lose weight it gets increasingly harder to lose additional weight. If this is the case, the solution is to increase your calorie deficit by either reducing your caloric intake or increasing your activity level – or both. This done you should once more see a more detectable weight loss each week.

The most probable cause for a real weight loss plateau, however, is that over time you have become careless, either eating slightly more, or exercising less, or both. Yet another cause could be temporary water retention as discussed in the preceding section. More than likely it is a combination of all of these factors that makes you believe you have stopped losing weight.

If you encounter a weight loss plateau, the first thing to do is sit back and analyze your eating and exercise patterns. A good technique is to keep a diet diary, honestly listing everything you eat and the associated calories. (Most people underestimate their caloric intake by at least 15 percent.) Add the calories consumed for a week and divide by seven to compute an average daily caloric intake. Then enter either Weight Maintenance Tables 40 or 41 at your current weight and activity level and determine your maintenance calories. Next, calculate your all-important daily caloric deficit (maintenance calories minus your daily caloric intake). Then make an estimate of your expected weekly weight loss by multiplying your daily caloric deficit by seven and dividing the result by 7700. This is illustrated in the following example.

Example: A relatively inactive 70-year-old woman weighs 60 kg on a 1500-kcal reducing diet feels that she has stopped losing weight, has reached a plateau. How should she proceed?

First, she conducts a careful review of her eating patterns and finds that her average daily intake is not 1500 kcalories but is actually closer to 1800 kcalories! Now we again temporarily jump ahead to Weight Maintenance **Table 42** on page 131 where she determines that at 60 kg her weight maintenance level is about 1947 kcalories per day. Her daily deficit then is only 1965 – 1800 = 165 kcalories. In one week she will lose a meager 165 x 7 / 7700 = 0.15 kilos!

So she is probably still losing weight, albeit so slowly that in the short term her assessment is that her weight loss has stopped and she has hit a mysterious weight-loss- blocking plateau. As a rule then, to avoid the perception that a dreaded weight loss plateau has been reached, you should not allow your deficit to fall below about 500 kcalories a day. This will assure a more observable weight loss of at least half a kilo per week.

Weight Loss Maxims

Once the parameters involved in weight loss are related in a mathematical equation, it is possible to state some principles or maxims. (It is also possible to deduce most of the following truisms by examining the Weight Loss Prediction tables.)

1) Given two people the same age, gender and activity level, and on the same reducing diet, **the heavier person will lose weight faster than the thinner person**. For instance, according to Table 25, on 1500 kcalories, it would take a relatively inactive 60 kg man 68 days to lose 5 kilos; whereas the same table indicates a man who weighs 100 kg would only take 30 days to lose 5 kilos.

2) Given two people the same age, gender and activity level, and on the same reducing diet (i.e., consuming the same number of calories), the **taller person will lose weight at a faster rate**.

3) Given a male and female, the same age, weight, activity level and on the same reducing diet, **the man will lose weight faster than the woman**. This is because women most often have less muscle mass and, therefore, lower basal metabolic rates than men.

4) Given two individuals, the same gender, weight and activity level, **the younger person will lose weight faster than the older person**. The lesson is if you are overweight start on a weight loss diet now because it will only become **more difficult to lose weight as you get older.**

5) It follows that if your **caloric intake is constant over the years you will slowly gain weight as you age.** This is because you naturally lose muscle and your basal metabolic rate decreases as you advance in age, and most people tend not to be as active as they get older.

6) If your **caloric intake on a weight-loss diet is constant, your rate of weight loss will decrease with time.** Hence, to lose weight at a constant rate over time, you must eat slightly less (or exercise harder) as you lose weight.

Which Weight Loss Diet?

Sure you want to lose weight but what diet should you choose? Low carb, high protein, low fat? Atkins, Zone, South Beach, Pritikin, or Ornish? What about the grapefruit diet or Sugar Busters? And on and on. Each fad diet that comes along promises to be the true path to weight loss.

In reality you can lose weight on almost any diet. Many of the aforementioned diets don't even mention the word calorie, but when analyzed carefully it's clear that by restricting certain foods these diets are in fact limiting calories. You lose weight when you eat fewer calories than your body burns. It doesn't matter whether the calories are from protein, carbohydrates or fat. Calories are calories.

Low-fat diets gained popularity in the 1990's. And you can lose weight on a low-fat diet provided you also lower your calorie intake. But in recent years, even the strictest fat-limiting advocates have to admit that not all fats are alike. Some fats are bad for you, but others are actually healthy and should be included in any diet – even a weight-loss diet.

Anecdotal evidence and weight loss research indicates that early on you will probably lose weight faster on a low-carb diet. The reason is two-fold. First at the start of any diet there is usually considerable loss of water – and water loss is particularly high for low-carb diets. But the main reason is that when you exclude carbohydrate-rich foods, you have no choice but to eat more fats and protein. Because fats and protein are digested more slowly than carbohydrates, most people don't feel quite as hungry on a low-carb reducing diet. So they eat less – eat fewer calories overall – and lose weight. The problem with low-carb diets is that they are nutritionally unsound and are difficult to stay with over the long haul. So what to do?

What Makes a Good Diet?

Every good weight-loss diet must have the following three characteristics:
1) A good diet must provide an understanding of weight control as well as the knowledge needed to reduce your weight to the desired level.
2) A good diet must help you remain healthy while you are losing weight.
3) A good diet must lead you to a healthier way of eating and exercising that will help you, in the long term, keep off the weight you have lost.

The weight-loss diet that fits these constraints is the so-called "balanced diet;" i.e., a diet that is not only low calorie but also nutritionally balanced.

Weight Loss Eating Patterns

Using the nutrition and weight loss information presented to this point, you should be able to plan a reducing diet suited to your individual likes and lifestyle. This offers great flexibility, but requires that you take care and use the **Guidelines for Healthy Eating** when choosing foods from all six-food groups.

After you determine your daily diet calorie allowance from the Weight Loss Prediction Tables, the next step is to decide on a weekly routine, i.e., how you will distribute your calories among the days of the week. As already mentioned your caloric allowance need not be the same for every day of the week. Next apportion your daily caloric allowance among the meals of the day according to your personal eating habits. The following approximate daily calorie distributions are suggestions only. (Feel free, however, to modify this calorie distribution to suit your eating routine and lifestyle.)

	900	1200	1500
Breakfast	200	200	250
Lunch	250	250	350
Dinner	450	670	780
Snacks	0	80	150

Suggested Daily Calorie Distribution

Set Meals for Calorie Control

Are you concerned about having to count calories? Whether on a reducing diet or trying to maintain your weight, allocating a specific number of calories for each meal makes it unnecessary to keep a running calorie tally for an entire day. Instead, you only need to monitor the number of calories eaten at each meal – and there are ways to keep even this to a minimum by utilizing a concept called "Set Meals" – a strategy not very different than the measured-food-to-eat systems used by diet plans such as Jenny Craig and NutriSystem. Except with the "Set Meals" system you control what you eat.

A Set Meal is a food serving where the ingredients vary - but is almost identical in calorie count and nutritional content day after day. Any meal during the day that is completely under your control is a Set Meal candidate.

For instance, suppose you prepare breakfast at home almost every day. Plan perhaps three set breakfasts. One might be based on cereal and fruit, another on eggs and toast, and so on. Variety is obtained by having more than one choice for a Set Meal, and by eating different kinds of cereal, or fruit, or egg preparations (scrambled, over easy, soft-boiled) – all within the same Set Meal. Once this is done, the number of calories in each of the Set Meal can be easily calculated. Then, try to plan set meals for lunch.

The more Set Meals you have in a day, the less calorie counting. If you have set meals for both breakfast and lunch, then you only have to

113

monitor dinner calories.

Despite all the information that has been provided here, if you would rather not go through the trouble of planning a personal diet routine, use one of the pre-planned 900, 1200, or 1500 kcal eating patterns shown in Tables 35 to 37. These dietary patterns are particularly recommended because they adhere to the U.S. Department of Agriculture Dietary Guidelines and are nutritionally sound.

Example: Devise a well-balanced, nutritious, weight-loss-eating plan for a 32-year-old woman who wants to start on a 1500-kcal diet. A married mother of two, she works full-time as a nurse on the day shift.

First she has to distribute her 1500 kcal among the meals of the day. Based on her eating habits, as a first pass she decides to allocate approximately 275 kcal for breakfast, 300 for lunch, 650 for dinner and 275 Calories for three snacks. (At this point, these calorie values are tentative and subject to alteration as her eating plan unfolds.)

Next, she has to establish her Set Meals, the meals she has control over, and also account for the foods she likes and dislikes. She certainly has control over breakfast, and she has decided to bring a lunch to the hospital rather than eat in the cafeteria. So she also has control over what she eats for lunch. When she gets home from work, she and her husband prepare dinner together and sometimes they eat out.

For breakfast she likes cereal with skim milk, or eggs and toast. For lunch she prefers things that are quick and easy to prepare like tuna fish, soup, cottage cheese, or cereal (if she hasn't already had cereal for breakfast). She also enjoys a morning and afternoon snack. Now we are ready to layout her meal plan for every day of the week.

Using these facts as input, she establishes the weight loss eating plan broadly outlined in Table 37. Next, she calculates the number of calories in the foods comprising her Set Meals, i.e., her breakfasts and lunches and snacks. The details behind Table 37 are in a spreadsheet (not shown because of size limitations).

For breakfast, "Cereal (M)" consists of a healthy cereal (such as Oat Meal, Wheatena, Farina, Shredded Wheat, Cheerios, Wheat Chex, Wheaties, and some Kashi cereals) with skim milk and topped with a half a banana or other fruit. "Cereal (Y)" substitutes non-fat yogurt for skim milk. In addition, 125 mL of fruit juice are part of every breakfast.

For lunch, acceptable soups include tomato, vegetable, pea, actually any soup where a serving is 125 kcal or less. Any low-calorie salad dressing (about 25 kcal per 15 mL) can be used. Remember to use tuna packed in water rather than oil. Worth noting is that every effort was made to nutritionally balance the meals in a given day. For example, either milk, yogurt or cottage cheese are present every day.

	Mon	Tues	Weds	Thurs	Fri	Sat	Sun
Morning Meal	Cereal (M)	Toast	Egg	Cereal (M)	Egg	Cereal (M)	Egg
Snack	Fruit	Yogurt & Fruit	Yogurt & Fruit	Fruit	Yogurt & Fruit	Fruit	Yogurt & Fruit
Afternoon Meal	Soup	Cereal (S)	Cereal (S)	Tuna	Cereal (S)	Tuna	Cereal (S)
Snack	Nuts & Seeds	Nuts & Seeds	Nuts & Seeds	Nuts & Seeds	Nuts & Seeds	Nuts & Seeds	Nuts & Seeds
kcalories	730	805	680	730	730	850	680

Table 37: Weight Loss Eating Plan

Overall variety is achieved by having different brands of cereal, different kinds of fruit, several types of nuts and seeds, different kinds of soup, and eggs prepared in various ways. To make sure she is getting the proper amount of nutrients every day, for dinner she plans to have at least two other vegetable servings, a starch (potato or brown rice), and a small serving of fish, poultry, lean meat, or a plant protein. Her evening snack (dessert) depends on the number of calories she has remaining after dinner. Dessert could be a small glass of skim milk and yes a cookie, or a low-calorie pudding, etc. Coffee or tea (with skim milk and an artificial sweetener if desired) can be served at any meal or as part of a snack.

From Table 37 we notice that her calorie total for breakfast, lunch and snacks is not the same for every day of the week. Because it is impractical to assign a different dinner calorie target for every day of the week, we average the daily totals for breakfast, lunch and snacks (as shown in the worksheet), and use the average value to calculate her allowable dinner calories. Table 37 indicates that for dinner (and any evening snack) she is allowed a total of 756 kcal (1500 kcal minus the calories she has already eaten for breakfast, lunch and day-time snacks).

This dinner calorie total should be relatively easy to stay within provided she eats well-balanced meals with portion sizes consistent with

115

her 756 kcal limit. To understand what "reasonable" portion sizes should look like for a 756-kcal meal, at first she will probably have to count calories at dinner. After a few weeks of counting dinner calories, however, she should be able to judge what is and what is not an acceptable portion size for the different foods on her plate – and then proceed without actually counting calories.

Using this Set Meal technique, she only has to judge or estimate her dinner calories to assure that she is close to her diet calorie allowance on a weekly basis. If you are uneasy about devising your own weight loss eating plan, either use the pre-planned diets in the next section, or seek the professional advice of a registered dietitian. Registered dietitians translate the science of nutrition into everyday information about food, and are trained to assist people with their individual diets and meal plans. Go online to find a registered dietitian in your area.

Finally, how should she manage the inevitable, i.e., when she has to attend a business luncheon, or an all-day business meeting, or she goes on a vacation? In other words, how should she handle those days when she just can't follow her weight loss eating plan? See **"Helpful Diet Strategies."** on page 122.

Pre-Planned Diets

Despite all the information that has been provided here, if you would rather not go through the trouble of planning a personal diet eating routine, use one of the pre-planned 900, 1200, or 1500 kcal eating patterns shown in Tables 38 to 40. The diets are recommended because they adhere to the U.S. Department of Agriculture Dietary Guidelines and are nutritionally sound.

Intentionally Left Blank

Morning Meal A	Morning Meal B	Morning Meal C
½ cup fruit or juice	½ cup fruit or juice	½ cup fruit or juice
30 g cereal	1 egg cooked w/o fat	30 g cereal
1 cup skim milk	1 slice dry toast	1 cup fat-free yogurt
Coffee or tea	Coffee or tea	Coffee or tea
Mid-Day Meal A	**Mid-Day Meal B**	**Mid-Day Meal C**
1 cup fat-free cheese	60 g lean meat	90 g fish
1 cup vegetables	1 cup vegetables	1 cup vegetables
Coffee or tea	1 slice bread	1 slice bread
	Coffee or tea	Coffee or tea
Evening Meal A	**Evening Meal B**	**Evening Meal C**
60 g Chicken	90 g fish	90 g Chicken
Green salad + dressing	Green salad + dressing	Green salad + dressing
1 slice bread	1 cup fat-free yogurt	1 slice bread
1 cup fruit	Coffee or tea	1 cup fruit
Coffee or tea		Water
905 kcal	**930 kcal**	**930 kcal**

Table 38: 900 kcal Diet Menus

Note: 1 cup = 250 mL (metric cup). 900-kcalorie reducing diet is only suitable for a small, relatively low-weight person who wants to lose a few extra kilos. **In most cases, a 900-kcalorie diet should be used only under a physician's supervision.**

Morning Meal A	Morning Meal B	Morning Meal C
½ cup fruit or juice	½ cup fruit or juice	½ cup fruit or juice
30 g cereal	1 egg cooked w/o fat	30 g cereal
1 cup skim milk	1 slice dry toast	1 cup fat-free yogurt
Coffee or tea	Coffee or tea	Coffee or tea
Mid-Day Meal A	**Mid-Day Meal B**	**Mid-Day Meal C**
1 cup fat-free cheese	60 g lean meat	120 g fish
1 cup vegetables	1 cup vegetables	1 cup vegetables
Coffee or tea	1 slice bread	1 slice bread
	Coffee or tea	Coffee or tea
Evening Meal A	**Evening Meal B**	**Evening Meal C**
100 g lean meat	120 g fish	120 g chicken
Green salad + dressing	Green salad + dressing	Green salad + dressing
1 cup vegetables	1 cup vegetables	1 medium potato
1 slice bread	1 slice bread	1 cup fruit
1 cup fruit	1 cup fruit	Coffee or tea
Coffee or tea	Coffee or tea	
1110 kcal	**1120 kcal**	**1125 kcal**

Table 39: 1200 kcal Diet Menus

Note: 1 cup = 250 mL (metric cup). **Elective Calorie Budget**: In addition to the above, 80 kcal may be used as desired for a snack - such as ½ cup non-fat ice cream, or for 15 g of peanut butter to spread on a slice of bread, etc.

Morning Meal A	Morning Meal B	Morning Meal C
½ cup fruit or juice	½ cup fruit or juice	½ cup fruit or juice
1 oz. (30 g) cereal	1 egg cooked w/o fat	1 oz. (30 g) cereal
1 cup skim milk	2 slices dry toast	1 cup fat-free yogurt
1 slice dry toast	Coffee or tea	1 slice dry toast
Coffee or tea		Coffee or tea
Mid-Day Meal A	**Mid-Day Meal B**	**Mid-Day Meal C**
1 cup fat-free cottage ch	60 g lean meat	120 g fish
1 cup vegetables	1 cup vegetables	1 cup vegetables
1 slice bread	1 slice bread	1 slice bread
1 cup fruit	1 cup fat-free yogurt	Coffee or tea
Coffee or tea	Coffee or tea	
Evening Meal A	**Evening Meal B**	**Evening Meal C**
100 g lean meat	150 g fish	150 g chicken
Green salad + dressing	Green salad + dressing	Green salad + dressing
1 cup vegetables	1 cup rice	1 medium potato
1 slice bread	1 cup vegetables	1 cup vegetables
1 cup fruit	1 cup fruit	1 cup fruit
Coffee or tea	Coffee or tea	Coffee or tea
1365 kcal	**1370 kcal**	**1340 kcal**

Table 40: 1500 kcal Diet Menus

Note: 1 cup = 250 mL (metric cup). **Elective Calorie Budget**: In addition to the above, 140 kcalories may be used as desired for a snack - such as ¾ cup low-fat ice cream, or for 15 g of peanut butter to spread on a slice of bread, etc.

Notice that Tables 38 through 40 contain no recipes. For instance, the 1,200 Calorie Balanced Diet shown in Table 40 specifies ½ cup of vegetables, but does not identify the kind of vegetables and gives no advice regarding how the vegetables should be prepared. This is because Tables 39 to 41 are general diet guidelines around which more specific meals and recipes can be planned to suit individual preferences and taste.

Again, if you are not sure you can devise your own weight loss eating plan, or the pre-planned diets in the next section are not to your liking, seek the professional help of a registered dietitian.

Pre-Planned Diets Notes

The following notes apply to the 900, 1200 and 1500 diets shown in Tables 38 to 40.

1) Cereal should be whole grain and preferably unsweetened. At the top of the list are Old-fashioned Oat Meal, Wheatena and Shredded Wheat. Among other reasonably healthy choices are Cheerios, Wheat Chex, Wheaties some Kashi cereals and Farina.

2) Bread may be either plain or toasted whole wheat, whole rye or pumpernickel. If desired, bread may be sprayed with a zero-calorie butter substitute.

3) Meat should be lean cuts with all visible fat trimmed. Poultry should be limited to chicken or turkey breasts (white meat and skinless).

4) An unlimited amount of green salad may be eaten, but the salad dressing should contain no more than 1 tbsp of vegetable oil (olive, canola, sunflower, safflower etcetera).

5) Potato should be baked or boiled and (if desired) served with a tbsp of non-fat sour cream, or sprayed with a zero-calorie butter substitute. Where rice is specified, brown or wild rice is recommended.

6) Use freely as desired: clear unsweetened coffee, clear unsweetened tea, water (with a squeeze of lemon section if desired), seltzer water, and diet soda.

7) Use freely as desired: clear soups w/o fat, bouillon, and seasonings such as mustard, cinnamon, dill, herbs, red and black pepper, curry, vinegar, lemon juice and sections, and dill and sour pickles.

Helpful Diet Strategies

Everyone needs strategies to help stay on the right-diet track. Here are a few time-tested dieting techniques that work.

1) Exchange equivalent foods for variety and prevent boredom.

2) To avoid "hidden calories," prepare simple foods cooked in an uncomplicated manner.

3) Get a good cookbook and a calorie reference.

4) Learn to estimate portion sizes.

5) Use Set Meals to make calorie control easy.

6) Handle occasional overeating by compensating.

7) Keep log of what you eat.

8) Use technology to monitor the calories you eat.
9) If it suits your lifestyle, follow a weekly rather a daily calorie allowance.
10) Handle special situations by temporarily going on weight maintenance.
11) Check your progress by graphing your weight loss.

Again all are discussed in some detail in the sections that follow. Choose the strategy (or strategies) that are right for you.

Exchanging Foods

To prevent a diet from becoming monotonous, after a few weeks try exchanging or substituting foods – a technique used by dieticians. Exchanging a food listed in a diet for another food with approximately equal caloric value and nutritional content is the foundation of a successful long-term diet. Substitution possibilities are almost endless but have to be done carefully.

The easiest substitutions are those within the same food group, such as exchanging one vegetable variety for another, or a glass of milk for a cup of yogurt. More sophisticated exchanges cross food groups.

Simple is Better

When on a diet simple is better. Why? Because simple, uncomplicated meals will usually contain fewer "hidden calories" than more elaborate dishes. For example, straightforward broiled fish with micro-waved vegetables makes a nutritious, quick, low-calorie dinner – with no "hidden calories." To add interest to foods without adding calories, season with spices and condiments.

Get a Good Cookbook & Calorie Ref

Acquire a good low-calorie cookbook. Make sure the recipes cover breakfast, lunch and dinner, and all the recipes contain nutritional information, especially the number of calories per serving. In addition, **obtain a comprehensive food calorie guide** such as the excellent U.S.D. A. Home and Garden Bulletin No. 72: "Nutritive Value of Foods," which is online and can be downloaded at no cost.

Estimating Portion Sizes

Whatever calorie counting scheme you use, another dilemma for dieters is judging portion size. It makes no sense to worry about whether to apportion 280 or 300 kcal per 100 grams for a cut of lean meat if you have no idea whether the portion you are planning to eat weighs 100 or 300 grams. You must learn to estimate portion sizes with reasonable accuracy. The best way to do this is to start by weighing and measuring the food you eat. After about a week or two, your eye should be adjusted to what 100 grams of meat or 150 grams of fish look like, and you can then discontinue weighing.

Incidentally, judging the weight of meat is one of the most important parts of many diets. As a guide, 100 grams of meat is about the size of a slice of bread 10 x 10 x ½ cm. And kcalorie tables always refer to meat that has been cooked and trimmed of visible fat and bone.

How to Handle Overeating

It's a fact of life that no matter how determined you are to abide by your daily calorie goal, life has a way of interfering. In real life, you probably will not be able to eat the same number of calories day after day. Maybe it's your social life that interferes. Maybe you have to attend a wedding reception. Maybe an unexpected occasion arises where you know you're going to go over your daily calorie allowance. What should you do?

The way to handle the inevitable overeating is by compensating. You compensate by estimating how far you have strayed from your weight-loss diet and then make amends at the next opportunity (usually the next meal or two) – by eating less.

For instance, let's say you have to attend a business luncheon. Further, assume the meal has been pre-ordered so you have no choice but to eat what's served. At some point toward the end of the meal, make a mental estimate of the number of calories you have eaten. Suppose, even though you tried to be careful, your estimate is about 850 kcal. If your normal Set Lunch is 450 kcal, you know you have over done it by approximately 400 kcal. That night at dinner you decide to have water instead of wine, to forgo your evening snack and to take a half hour after-dinner walk. By doing this, before the end of the day, you will have compensated for the extra 400 kcal you ate at lunch.

Eating in Restaurants: To eat as few calories as possible, during your weight-loss diet adhere to the following restaurant guidelines. First, for an appetizer order fruit juice or melon. For your main course order broiled fish, poultry or a lean cut of meat cooked as plainly as possible (no butter, stuffing, gravy). Order steamed vegetables and maybe a baked potato. Have your salad with the dressing on the side. Finally, ask for fruit for dessert – or have just coffee or tea.

Keep a Log of What You Eat

Behavior research indicates that dieters who keep a record of what they eat generally have more successful outcomes. How should you go about this? Keep a food log.

You can keep your daily food log in a small notebook, a daily planner, a handheld organizer, your laptop, or Smart Phone, whatever works best for you. You should record the date, meal, food eaten, amount, calorie estimate, total calories for the day and any comments. To approximate the weight of a portion or serving use either a small scale or visually estimate the weight by employing rules of thumb, such as four ounces of meat or fish is about the size of a deck of cards, and one and one-half ounces of cheese is similar in size to a pair of dice. Once you know the weight, use either Table 22 (page 89), "Calorie Rank (per 100 gm) of Common Foods," or a more comprehensive calorie reference to determine the calories in a particular portion.

Diet Tip: The secret to a healthy weight loss diet is to make every calorie count in terms of your nutritional needs.

Handling Special Situations

Suppose you are in the middle of your diet and you have to travel overseas for a few weeks, or you have to leave on a planned three-week family vacation. In both circumstances you know you will never be able to resist the food and stay on your diet. What to do?

One solution is to go off your diet – temporarily. Essentially go on weight maintenance and try to at least return from your trip or vacation without having gained any weight. (Weight Maintenance is covered in the next chapter where you will learn how many calories you can eat to neither gain nor lose weight.) When you get back, you can pick up where you left off – back on your diet and resume your weight loss.

Plot Your Weight Loss

Another technique to help you track your weight loss progress, is to graphically compare your actual weight loss to your expected weight loss from the Weight Loss Prediction table that applies to you. If you're computer savvy you can plot your weight loss on your computer using a graphical software package. Otherwise, just use ordinary graph paper. Either way proceed as follows.

First, from the Weight Loss Prediction Table appropriate for your gender, age, and activity level, choose your diet calorie level. Next, using the data in the table, plot your predicted weight loss versus time on the diet. Draw a solid line through the data points. This is your baseline against which you will compare your actual weight loss. Weigh in at the start of your diet. Then, once a week, weigh yourself first thing in the morning and plot the value. If your weight loss is less than the predicted values, most likely you are either 1) cheating (eating more than your diet calorie allowance), or you're not as active as you think, as the weight loss prediction table you're using requires – or both.

Can You Target Weight Loss?

As you gain weight, a host of factors, the most important of which are genetics, gender, and age, determine where on your body you will put down fat. Let's say you have a particular area that's collected a lot of fat and it's bothering you – maybe it's around your abdomen (belly fat), your thighs or under your chin. Is there anything you can do to eliminate or just reduce the amount of fat in a particular annoying area? **The short answer is no**, but read on.

Losing Belly Fat

The truth of the matter is that your body decides where to put fat on and where to remove it, a system that is largely determined by your genetics. Your body distributes fat based on tactics developed over the eons.

Fat is stored in your abdomen, hips or buttocks because it takes less energy to carry fat accumulated in your midsection than other areas of your body. Keep in mind fat storage is a survival strategy, so your body tends to maximize energy efficiency in the formation, storage and use of body fat. Then, from an anthropological viewpoint, the location of body fat has reproductive implications. In women, fat is stored in the hips, buttocks and breasts to create a more attractive body in order to attract a potential mate. Lastly, your body amasses fat where you have put down fat cells when you were young.

Getting rid of abdominal fat has, undoubtedly, as great a level of misunderstanding as any weight loss subject. The major fallacy is that you can get rid of abdominal fat by working your abdominal muscles. This is based on the incorrect belief that fat is eliminated from a part of your body if you engage the muscles underneath that layer of fat. No such luck.

Last On First Off

This **general weight-change rule (based on observation) is "last on first off."** Assume as you gained weight, the first place you noticed it was on your thighs, next your buttocks, then your face. As you lose weight, it generally will come off in the reverse order, first from your face, then your rear and finally your thighs. And there is not much you can do about that. The truth is there is no food, no exercise, no magic belt, and no pill that will cause your body to lose fat in one place rather than another.

For women, this means the last place you're likely to lose fat is on your hips and buttocks. You may have already observed this phenomenon if you've ever been on a diet, or if you've lost weight but couldn't seem to lose that last bit of "stubborn" body fat.

For men, abdominal fat is probably the last fat that will disappear from your body. In the most likely progression, first you will lose fat from your face and extremities, such as your arms and legs, then from your upper torso, your chest, upper thighs and buttocks, and finally the fat stored in your abdomen. And science has not devised a technique to alter this fat reduction pattern.

So if you are really serious about getting rid of that abdominal fat, you're going to have to take a whole-body approach – and get used to the idea that belly fat is likely to be the last fat to go. This isn't what you want to hear, but it's the truth. To reduce body fat, you need to start consuming fewer calories than you expend on a daily basis. In other words, you need a calorie deficit. In time, your body will start converting fat into useable energy, and by doing so, fat stores will begin to disappear all across your body. But fat won't just magically vanish from one targeted place.

If you follow a healthy weight-loss diet combined with aerobic exercise and strength training, you will lose weight and eventually that weight loss will eliminate or reduce your particular problem area. In summary, despite what you may have read, there is no diet regimen or exercise routine that can "target" a particular area of your body. Just be patient and as you lose weight that problem area will eventually disappear.

Words of Caution

A reducing diet is best supervised by a physician. This is especially true when a great deal of weight needs to be lost, or if you have an ailment or a history of medical problems. The Weight Loss Prediction tables cover a wide range of possibilities. And while the values in the tables are theoretically attainable, they are not necessarily recommended for everyone. In some cases the wide ranges were computed and included for completeness.

Most physicians recommend that weight loss should be limited to no more than one to two pounds per week, except for very large individuals, or if the total amount of weight to be lost is very small. In these cases, an acceptable weight loss rate may be as high as three pounds per week. And many nutritionists feel that weight-loss diets should not have food intakes below 900 to 1200 kcal. This is because it is difficult to obtain the proper amount of essential nutrients below these levels.

Don't Give Up!

Finally, realize that, in all likelihood, the road to your weight loss goal will not be an easy one. You didn't gain all that extra weight last week, did you? No, of course not. You probably accumulated the extra weight over the course of several years. No doubt it was a slow, gradual change that occurred because your daily caloric intake during that time exceeded your daily caloric expenditure by some small amount. The point is that small but permanent changes in your diet can put you back on track and create the permanent weight loss you desire.

Don't get frazzled if you have a few setbacks along the way. Many dieters think that if they have a weekend or even a week where they eat more than they should, they might as well give up. Not true. Many successful dieters have lots of bad days. But they don't expect to be perfect. When you hit a bump in the road, simply take a break, relax, and re-start your diet. Successful dieters know that losing weight is a journey – with good days and some bad days – all are expected as they proceed along the road toward their weight loss goal.

WEIGHT MAINTENANCE

Within five years, more than 90 percent of all dieters regain every pound they have lost. Why? In most instances it is because after losing weight most people eventually revert to their pre-diet eating and exercising habits, and this inevitably leads to their regaining the weight they lost – and often more. The fact is the less we weigh, the less we need to eat to sustain that lower weight. The quantity of food energy required to <u>maintain</u> a particular weight is again a function of sex, age, weight and activity level, as is clearly shown in Weight Maintenance Tables 41 and 42 (on pages 130 and 131).

Weight Maintenance Example

Consider a 63-year-old relatively inactive woman who weighed 90 kilos at the start of her reducing diet. After losing 20 kilos, she weighed 70 kilos. Determine her weight maintenance calories before and after she lost weight. Determine her weight maintenance calories before and after she lost weight.

From **Table 42** (page 131) find that before she started her diet, when she weighed 90 kilos, her weight maintenance level was 2622 kcal, meaning she must have been eating about 2688 kcal of food per day. After her diet, the same table shows that in order to maintain her lower weight of 70 kilos she must restrict her food intake in the future to 2243 kcal per day. On average, then, to neither gain nor lose weight at 70 kilos she must consume about 379 kcal per day less than she did when she weighed 90 kilos.

This person could help her cause by engaging in some form of exercise everyday. For example, if she walked 45 minutes every day at moderate 5.5 kph pace (covering a distance of slightly more than 4 kilometers), she could eat an additional (305 – 90) x 45 / 60 = 161 kcalories per day without gaining weight. (See Table 9 on page 32.)

Weight Control - Life-Long Battle

A study, published in a 2005 issue of the Annals of Internal Medicine, that followed 4000 people for three decades suggests that in the long term, 90 percent of men and 70 percent of women will become overweight (with a $BMI \geq 25$). Interestingly, half of the men and women in the study, who had made it well into adulthood without a weight problem, ultimately also became overweight and a third became obese (with a $BMI \geq 30$). The message is that you can never become complacent. **You must continually watch your weight because we are all at risk of becoming overweight.**

When you reach your mid to late twenties, you slowly start to lose muscle and add fat as part of the natural aging process. But muscle is

Weight Maintenance Calories For Men

Weight kg.	Age: 51-65 years			Age: 66-80 years		
	Sedent*	Inactive*	Active*	Sedent*	Inactive*	Active*
54	1954	2038	2224	1865	1949	2136
56	19985	2081	2275	1904	1991	2185
58	2035	2125	2326	1943	2033	2234
60	2075	2168	2375	1982	2075	2282
62	2114	2210	2425	2020	2116	2331
64	2153	2252	2474	2058	2157	2378
66	2192	2294	2523	2095	2197	2426
68	2230	2336	2571	2132	2238	2473
70	2268	2377	2619	2169	2277	2520
75	2362	2478	2737	2260	2376	2635
80	2453	2577	2854	2348	2472	2749
85	2543	2675	2969	2436	2567	2861
90	2632	2771	3083	2521	2661	2972
95	2719	2866	3195	2606	2753	3082
100	2805	2959	3305	2689	2844	3190
105	2889	3052	3415	2771	2934	3297
110	2973	3143	3524	2853	3023	3404
115	3055	3233	3631	2933	3111	3509
120	3137	3323	3738	3112	3198	3613
125	3218	3411	3844	3091	3284	3717
130	3297	3499	3949	3168	3370	3820

Table 41 Weight Maintenance Calories-Men

* Relatively Inactive has been shortened to Inactive and Moderately Active has been shortened to Active.

Weight Maintenance Calories For Women

Weight kg.	Age: 51-65 years			Age: 66-80 years		
	Sedent*	Inactive*	Active*	Sedent*	Inactive*	Active*
46	1674	1745	1904	1605	1676	1835
48	1715	1789	1955	1644	1719	1885
50	1755	1832	2005	1684	1761	1934
52	1795	1875	2055	1722	1803	1983
54	1834	1918	2105	1760	1844	2031
56	1873	1960	2154	1798	1885	2079
58	1911	2001	2202	1835	1925	2126
60	1950	2042	2250	1872	1965	2173
62	1987	2083	2298	1909	2005	2220
64	2024	2124	2345	1945	2044	2266
66	2061	2164	2392	1981	2083	2312
68	2098	2203	2439	2017	2122	2357
70	2134	2243	2485	2052	2160	2403
75	2224	2340	2600	2139	2255	2515
80	2312	2436	2712	2225	2348	2625
85	2398	2530	2824	2309	2440	2734
90	2483	2622	2934	2391	2531	2842
95	2566	2714	3042	2473	2620	2949
100	2649	2804	3150	2553	2708	3054
110	2811	2981	3362	2711	2881	3262
120	2969	3154	3570	2865	3051	3466

Table 42 Weight Maintenance Calories-Women

* Relatively Inactive has been shortened to Inactive and Moderately Active has been shortened to Active.

metabolically active tissue. This means your muscles use calories when they work, as well as when they repair and refuel. Fat, on the other hand, requires very few calories to exist. This is one of the reasons you need fewer calories to remain at the same weight as you get older.

In weight maintenance, it is the number of calories you eat over the long term that is important. As an illustration, the weight maintenance value of 2243 kcal per day for the 63-year-old woman in the previous example amounts to about 818700 kcal in a single year. Now realize that an annual error of only two percent of this total (that is roughly 16400 kcal per year, or 45 kcal per day) would result in a weight gain of more than two kilos in one year, and the importance of knowing and adhering to your personal weight maintenance calorie value becomes apparent. In brief, **to control your weight it is the number of calories eaten over the long term that matters**.

Obviously, it would be impossible for the woman in the previous example to eat exactly 2243 kcal day after day. Errors are inevitable and experience has shown that when people err they do so on the high side. They consume more calories than their maintenance value, rarely less. To allow for occasional overeating or days when you can't exercise, plan to eat about seven percent below the values in the maintenance tables, or for the female in the example about 2080 kcal per day rather than the 2243 kcal shown in the weight maintenance table – leaving her room for an occasional calorie splurge, or a missed exercise session.

Planning Maintenance Eating

Once you are at your "best weight," or achieve a weight you are comfortable with, maintenance begins. Weight maintenance is in fact more difficult than being on a weight-loss diet. Why? Chiefly because maintenance requires a life-long commitment, a commitment to a new life style where you eat balanced nutritious meals that are within your maintenance calorie allowance.

Any motivational speech made at this point isn't going to be much help five and ten years down the road – when I trust you will still be in maintenance mode. Understand that if you really want to keep off the weight you have lost you will have to practice a good deal of self-discipline for a long time. Even the well motivated, however, need a good plan to succeed. The following approach (which is very similar to that discussed in the preceding "Planning Weight Loss Eating Patterns") is recommended:
1) Use Table 41 or 42 (for senior men and women) to determine your daily weight-maintenance calorie allowance.

2) Then decide on a weekly routine, i.e., how your calorie allowance is to be distributed among the days of the week. (As stated previously our caloric intake need not be the same for every day of the week.)

3) Next allocate the daily caloric allowance among the meals of the day according to your eating habits.

Obviously, a detailed meal plan for every possible calorie level cannot be included here, but given the information covered so far it should be possible to plan eating patterns you can live with for any weight maintenance calorie allowance. (See the example that follows immediately). Granted this will take some work but in the long run it will be time well spent.

Maintenance Plan Example

Devise a weight maintenance eating plan for a 58-year-old man who, after losing 10 kilos, weighs 68 kg. He describes his activity level as moderately actively. An engineering consultant, he works out of an office in his home.

First, from Table 41 (page 130), we find that at 68 kg his maintenance level is 2571 kcal. To determine how many kcalories per day he should plan to consume, we deduct seven percent from 2571 to allow for occasional overeating (or under-exercising). The result is about 2390 kcal per day – the number of calories he should plan on eating most days.

Then, we have to establish the meals he has control over (these will be his Set Meals), and also account for the foods he likes and dislikes. Because on most days he is home all day, he has control over every meal except the evening meal. (When his wife gets home from work, they prepare the evening meal together or sometimes go out to eat.)

We will assume that for his morning meal the man in this example likes cereal (with skim or soy milk) or eggs, and for his afternoon meal he prefers a tuna sandwich, soup or cereal (if he has not already had cereal for his morning meal). He also enjoys a morning and afternoon snack. Now he is ready to layout his meal plan for every day of the week. His resulting maintenance eating plan is broadly outlined in Table 41. Next, he calculates the number of Calories in the foods comprising his Set Meals, i.e., his breakfasts and mid-day meals and snacks. Again, the details behind Table 43 are in a spreadsheet (not shown here because of size limitations).

	Mon	Tues	Weds	Thurs	Fri	Sat	Sun
Morning Meal	Cereal (M)	Toast	Egg	Cereal (M)	Egg	Cereal (M)	Egg
Snack	Fruit	Yogurt & Fruit	Yogurt & Fruit	Fruit	Yogurt & Fruit	Fruit	Yogurt & Fruit
Afternoon Meal	Soup	Cereal (S)	Cereal (S)	Tuna	Cereal (S)	Tuna	Cereal (S)
Snack	Nuts& Seeds	Nuts & Seeds	Nuts & Seeds	Nuts& Seeds	Nuts & Seeds	Nuts& Seeds	Nuts & Seeds
Evening kcalories	1175	955	1075	1100	1075	1100	1075

Table 43: Sample Maintenance Eating Plan

As shown in Table 43, Cereal (M) indicates a cereal mix with skim milk, and that four ounces of juice are included with every breakfast choice. Worth noting is the fact that he made an effort to balance his meals within a given day. For example, he uses skim milk in his breakfast cereal and soy milk in the cereal he eats at lunch. Thus either skim milk or yogurt are present every day. **Overall variety is achieved by having different brands of cereal, different kinds of fruit, several types of nuts and seeds, different soup, and eggs prepared in various ways.** To assure he is getting the proper amount of nutrients every day, for his evening meal he always intends to have a large salad, at least two other vegetable servings, a starch (potato or brown rice), and a small serving of fish, poultry, lean meat, or a plant protein. His evening snack (dessert) always includes a glass of skim milk and yes a few cookies. (Nobody is perfect!)

For his evening meal, his calorie allowance is his Maintenance Calories minus the Calories he has already eaten for breakfast, mid-day meal and snacks. However, from Table 43 we notice that his Calorie total for breakfast, mid-day meal and snacks is not the same for every day of the week. This is not unexpected.

Because it is impractical to assign a different evening meal Calorie target for every day of the week, we average the daily totals for breakfast, mid-day meal and snacks (as shown in the worksheet), and use the average value to calculate the allowable calories for his evening meal. From Table 43 we see that he is allowed roughly 1000 kcal for his evening meal.

This evening meal calorie total should satisfy the appetite of the man in the example and should be easy to stay within provided he eats well-balanced meals with "reasonable" portion sizes. To understand what "reasonable" portion sizes should look like for a 1000-kcal meal, at first he will probably have to count calories at his evening meal. After a few weeks of counting evening meal calories, however, he should be able to judge what is and what is not an acceptable portion size for the different foods on his plate – without actually counting calories.

Using this technique, the he only has to judge or estimate his evening meal calories to assure that he is close to his maintenance Calories on a weekly basis. This plan should make it easier for him to control what he eats and maintain his new lower weight over the long haul. Once again, if you are not sure you can devise your own weight maintenance eating plan, seek the professional advice of a registered dietitian.

How should he manage the inevitable, i.e., when he has to attend an all-day business meeting, or he goes on a vacation? In other words, how should he handle those days when he just can not follow his weight maintenance eating plan? First of all, he knows that his maintenance eating pattern is approximately 400 kcal for breakfast, 500 kcal for the mid-day meal, 200 kcal for snacks, 1000 kcal for the evening meal and 250 kcal for dessert. And if he has been following this pattern for some time, he should be able to recognize the kinds of food and the amounts (portion sizes) that make up the calories he is allowed at each meal. Then with the added understanding of how to estimate the calorie content of various foods, he should be able to eat meals that approximate the calorie content of his weight maintenance eating plan. Lastly, if this approach does not work for him, he should realize that a day or two off his maintenance eating regimen is not the end of the world.

Mini Diets Maintain Weight Loss

Some people go through life maintaining their weight without thinking about how much they eat or exercise. When they occasionally eat a bigger meal, they seem to automatically eat less at the next meal or they exercise more, or they do both. If for some reason they expend more energy, they instinctively eat more. These people are able to maintain an almost constant weight without any effort. For most of us, however, weight control is more difficult, and we must be vigilant. For us weight control is a relentless life-long challenge.

When on a weight-loss diet, check and record your progress by weighing yourself at the same time two or three days per week. Once you are in weight maintenance mode, i.e., you have reached your desired weight level, weigh in about once a week. Small, natural weight fluctuations can be ignored, but action is called for if you experience a "noteworthy" increase in weight.

What is a noteworthy weight gain? For a 60-kg person a two kilo increase would be noteworthy; whereas for a 100-kg individual a five-kilo weight gain would be noteworthy. Both would signal a call to action. Incidentally, for most people, over a lifetime, noteworthy weight shifts are all but inevitable. Nevertheless, you should consider a noteworthy weight change a warning that you may be losing control of your weight and that you need to intervene to head off a potentially significant weight gain.

If you need to lose two or five kilos to get back to your best weight, go on a short-term mini diet. Revisit the Weight Loss Prediction tables and determine the calorie level needed to lose about one kilo per week. For example, a 60-year-old moderately active woman who weighs 60 kg on a 1200-kcal diet, should be able to lose two kilos in approximately 16 days, and a 60-year-old moderately active 100 kg man should be able to lose five kilos in approximately 29 days on a 1800-kcal diet.

Once back to your best weight, revisit and analyze your weight maintenance eating and exercise routines and make any adjustments needed to keep your weight on track. Furthermore, appreciate that in order to maintain a proper weight level you may have to go on a number of short-term mini diets over your lifetime to correct small weight maintenance calorie eating errors.

LIFE-LONG FITNESS

There are lots of reasons to get fit: a longer life expectancy, less illness, a healthful appearance, the ability to work (and play) with vigor and an energy reserve for emergencies. To repeat what was said earlier, people who undertake a physical fitness program and attain a heightened level of fitness, report a dramatic reduction in chronic fatigue, an improved ability to relax, more energy for day-to-day tasks, firmer muscles and increased strength. In short, they feel better and look better too!

Why then is it so easy to become a dropout when fitness offers such wonderful health benefits? A fitness plan may be the missing link to getting and staying fit. One of my early mentors, Dr. Kanaar was a wonderful swimmer. He not only taught me to be a more efficient swimmer, but at the same time he convinced me that it was especially **important for an individual starting a physical fitness program to set goals, have a plan and keep a fitness log.**

Everyone's personal goals and plan of attack will be different. Let us assume your goals are to lose 10 kilos and improve your overall health and fitness. First, commit yourself and start immediately. (Buy a notebook, or use your laptop or Smart phone because you will need to put your goals and plans in writing.) Next, plan how you are going to attain these goals. Broadly speaking, your overall plan might be to stop smoking; to begin a weight loss diet; and to start exercising. You must, however, be more specific and develop a detailed plan that indicates the when and how you are going to stop smoking, lose weight, etc. You might make up your mind to stop "cold turkey," or to enter a smoking secession program. Note the date you plan to start and the date you expect to be smoke free. Put it in writing!

For the weight loss portion of your plan, decide if you are going to go it alone or join some sort of clinical or non-clinical program. [All the information you need for a do-it-yourself weight loss program is in this book.] If you settle on a do-it-yourself program, again note the diet calorie level, milestone dates for weight loss, etc. Put it in writing!

Then choose an exercise routine. Again using the principles covered in this book devise a realistic plan with time, place, type of exercise and frequency. Put it writing!

By now you must appreciate why you need a notebook (or use your Smart phone, or laptop). Once you actually start implementing your plan, you should also keep an exercise log and a food log to record your progress. An all-in-one fitness log that includes exercise as well as food is a good idea. As you progress, periodically update your fitness plan. Enlist the support of your family and friends and do not forget to reward yourself when you reach a milestone – for a job well done!

Keys to Life-Long Fitness

As with most pursuits, the earlier in life you begin the better. But regardless of your age, the sooner you start a fitness program the easier it will be to get in shape and the more time you will have to reap the benefits. So for less illness, for a longer life expectancy, for a healthful appearance, start on the path to physical fitness now!

Despite all the detailed information presented in this book the path to life-long fitness is actually deceptively simple, and can be reduced to five basic keys. Assuming you have had a medical checkup, the five basic keys to life-long fitness are:

Key 1: Stop smoking and limit the consumption of alcoholic beverages. For some this will be difficult but both are absolutely necessary for life-long fitness.

Key 2: Keep your weight under control. Know your maintenance calorie value, i.e., how many calories you can eat to neither gain nor lose weight. Periodically you might experience a noteworthy weight gain. If this happens go on a mini-diet.

Key 3: Practice good nutrition by eating a variety of foods from each food group – all within your caloric allowance.

Key 4: Engage in some form of moderate strength training at least two non-consecutive days per week. Try to also get in some balance-training exercises – if you decide you need them.

Key 5: Engage in some form of moderate aerobic exercise every single day of the year. That is right every day! (If need be, cut back your aerobic workout on the days you do your strength exercises.)

To repeat, make every effort to engage in some form of moderate aerobic exercise every single day of the year! And try to exercise at the same time every day. This will probably mean rearranging priorities and putting exercise close to the top of your list. Soon exercise will become a part of your daily routine and you will not feel right unless you have had your daily run, or daily walk, etc.

Sure, there will be some days when it may seem impossible to fit exercise into your hectic schedule. Everyone would like to be able to workout for an uninterrupted hour, but the good news is that studies have shown that workouts as short as 15 minutes can improve your health. So on those very hectic, crazy days, try to fit in several 15-minute workouts whenever you can. Do the best with the time you have. Any other occasional additional exercise such as a round of golf on the weekend, a game of handball, cross-country skiing, attending a yoga class, is fine, beneficial, but should be considered secondary to your daily aerobic workout.

Make It Happen

At this point, you have everything you need to succeed. You have an understanding of the fundamentals of exercise, nutrition and weight control. You have set realistic fitness goals, and you have a good fitness plan. If you combine all these with intense desire you'll be unstoppable. Your fitness regimen will work wonders and will have you looking and feeling better both physically and mentally. And when you reach your goals and look and feel your best, your spirit will soar.

NoPaperPress eBooks and Paperbacks

100-Day Super Diet-1200 Cal*
100-Day Super Diet-1500 Cal*
100-Day No-Cooking Diet-1200 Cal*
100-Day No-Cooking Diet-1500 Cal*
90-Day Smart Diet-1200 Cal*
90-Day Smart Diet-1500 Cal*
90-Day No-Cooking Diet - 1200 Cal*
90-Day No-Cooking Diet - 1500 Cal*
90-Day Perfect Diet - 1200 Cal*
90-Day Perfect Diet - 1500 Cal*
60-Day Perfect Diet-1200 Cal*
60-Day Perfect Diet-1500 Cal*
50-Day Flex Diet-1200 Cal*
50-Day Flex Diet-1500 Cal*
30-Day Quick Diet - Women*
30-Day Quick Diet for Men*
30-Day No-Cooking Diet*
30-Day Diet - Women - Metric*
30-Day Diet for Men - Metric*
25 Day Easy Diet-1200 Cal*
25 Day Easy Diet-1500 Cal*
25-Day No-Cooking Diet
10-Day Express Diet
10-Day No-Cooking Diet*
7-Day Diet for Women*
7-Day Diet for Men*
7-Day No-Cooking Diets*
90-Day Gluten-Free Diet-1200 Cal*
90-Day Gluten-Free Diet-1500 Cal*
30-Day Gluten-Free Quick Diet*
30-Day Gluten-Free No-Cooking Diet*
7-Day Diet for Women - Metric*
7-Day Diet for Men - Metric
7-Day Gluten-Free Express Diet*
7-Day Gluten-Free No-Cooking Diet*
90-Day Vegetarian Diet-1200 Cal*
90-Day Vegetarian Diet-1500 Cal*
30-Day Vegetarian Diet*
7-Day Vegetarian Diet*
Weight Loss for Women*
Weight Loss for Women - Metric
Weight Loss for Women - UK
Weight Loss for Men*
Maximum Weight Loss - 1200 Cal*
Maximum Weight Loss - 1500 Cal*

Weight Loss for Men - Metric*
Maximum Weight Loss- 1200 Cal*
Maximum Weight Loss- 1500 Cal*
Weight Control - U.S. Edition*
Weight Control - Metric. Edition
Prof Weight Control Women - U.S.
Prof Weight Control Women - Metric
Prof Weight Control Men - U.S.
Prof Weight Control Men - Metric
Weight Maintenance - U.S. Ed*
Weight Maintenance - Metric. Ed*
Weight Maintenance - UK Ed
Weight Loss for Senior Men*
Weight Loss for Senior Women*
Eat Smart - U.S. Edition*
Eat Smart - Metric Edition
30-Day Mediterranean Diet
Exercise Smart - U.S. Edition*
Exercise Smart - Metric Edition
Exercise Smart - UK Edition*
Total Fitness - U.S. Edition
Total Fitness - Metric Edition
Total Fitness - UK Edition
Total Fitness for Women-U.S. Ed*
Total Fitness for Women - Metric
Total Fitness for Women - UK Ed
Total Fitness for Men - U.S. Ed*
Total Fitness for Men- Metric Ed*
Total Fitness for Men - UK Ed
Senior Fitness - U.S. Edition*
Senior Fitness - Metric Edition*
Senior Fitness - UK Edition*
Computer Diet - U.S. Edition*
Computer Diet - Metric Ed*
Reliable Weight Loss - U.S. Ed
101 Weight Loss Tips*
101 Healthy Eating Tips*
101 Lifelong Fitness Tips*
101 Weight Maintenance Tips
101 Weight Loss Recipes
101 GF Weight Loss Recipes
101 Veggie Weight Loss Recipes*
30-Day Mediterranean Diet*
90-Day Mediterranean Diet - 1200 Cal*
90-Day Mediterranean Diet - 1500 Cal*

* These titles are available as both ebooks and paperbacks. Our ebooks are sold by Amazon, Apple, Google, Barnes & Noble and Kobo, but our paperbacks are only sold by Amazon.

Vincent W. Antonetti, Ph.D. is an emeritus professor at Manhattan College in New York City. He is a weight control and fitness expert who 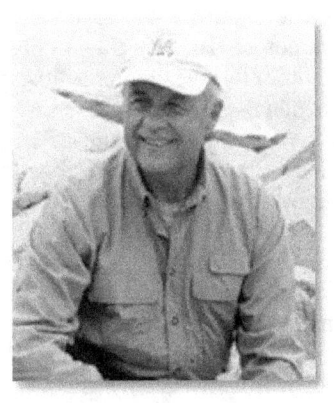 has lectured on fitness at IBM Management and Professional Development classes and often speaks on fitness and weight control. Among his many publications is his highly regarded "The Equations Governing Weight Change in Human Beings," published in the prestigious American Journal of Clinical Nutrition. This paper was the first to describe an accurate equation to calculate weight loss. Dr. Antonetti's critically acclaimed book The Computer Diet was given Consumer Guide magazine's highest recommendation. Recently, Dr. Antonetti coauthored "A Computational Tool to Simulate Energy Balance Components in Pharmacological Interventions," presented at Obesity Week 2016. He also co-authored (with Professor Diana Thomas) "Dynamic Modeling of Energy Expenditure to Estimate Dietary Energy Intake," Chapter 12 in Advances in the Assessment of Dietary Intake, published July 2017 by CRC Press.

Professor Antonetti is a life long exercise and nutrition enthusiast. Although a senior citizen he still maintains a vigorous physical fitness program - and has managed to maintain his weight to within 2 lbs (about one kg) of the 154 lbs (70 kg) it was when he graduated from college many years ago.

Disclaimer

This book offers general exercise, meal planning, nutrition and weight control information. It is not a medical manual and the author does not claim to be medically qualified. The material in this book is not intended to be a substitute for medical counseling. Every senior should have a medical checkup before beginning a physical fitness program. Every senior should have a medical checkup before beginning a fitness program (whether the program involves weight loss, nutritional changes, or exercise). Moreover, the physician conducting the medical exam should be made aware of and should approve the specific physical fitness routine planned. Further, the reader is cautioned that all fitness programs include some risk of injury or illness. Additionally, while the author and publisher have made every effort to ensure the accuracy of the information in this book, they make no representations or warranties regarding its accuracy or completeness. Further, neither the author nor publisher assume liability for any medical problems that might result from applying the methods in this book, or for any loss of profit, or any other commercial damages, including but not limited to special, incidental, consequential or other damages, and any such liability is hereby expressly disclaimed.

www.ingramcontent.com/pod-product-compliance
Lightning Source LLC
Chambersburg PA
CBHW060356290526
45791CB00002B/532